Children in Family Therapy: Treatment and Training

THE *JOURNAL OF PSYCHOTHERAPY & THE FAMILY* SERIES:

- *Computers and Family Therapy*

- *Divorce Therapy*

- *Family Therapy Education and Supervision*

- *Marriage and Family Enrichment*

- *Treating Incest: A Multiple Systems Perspective*

- *Depression in the Family*

- *The Use of Self in Therapy*

- *The Family Life of Psychotherapists: Clinical Implications*

- *Chronic Disorders and the Family*

- *Women, Feminism and Family Therapy*

- *Circumplex Model: Systemic Assessment and Treatment of Families*

- *Family Myths: Psychotherapy Implications*

- *Aging and Family Therapy: Practitioner Perspectives on Golden Pond*

- *Children in Family Therapy: Treatment and Training*

Children
in Family Therapy:
Treatment and Training

Joan J. Zilbach
Editor

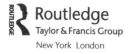
Routledge
Taylor & Francis Group
New York London

Children in Family Therapy: Treatment and Training has also been published as *Journal of Psychotherapy & the Family*, Volume 5, Numbers 3/4 1989.

First published 1989 by The Haworth Press, Inc.

Published 2020 by Routledge
52 Vanderbilt Avenue, New York, NY 10017
2 Park Square, Milton Park, Abingdon, Oxon OX14 4RN

Routledge is an imprint of the Taylor & Francis Group, an informa business

Library of Congress Cataloging-in-Publication Data

Children in family therapy : treatment and training / Joan J. Zilbach, editor.
    p. cm.
"Has also been published as Journal of psychotherapy & the family, volume 5, numbers 3/4, 1989" — T.p. verso.
    Includes bibliographies.
    ISBN 0-86656-774-7
    1. Family psychotherapy. 2. Child psychotherapy. I. Zilbach, Joan J., 1927-
RC488.5.C465   1989
616.89' 156 — dc20   89-32180
                                                                                          CIP

ISBN 13: 978-0-86656-774-9 (hbk)

Children in Family Therapy: Treatment and Training

CONTENTS

ABOUT THE EDITOR

Joan J. Zilbach, MD, is affiliated with the Fielding Institute in Santa Barbara, California, through which she teaches theories of marriage and family therapy with an emphasis on children. Dr. Zilbach is also currently in the private practice of family/couple therapy and psychoanalysis in Brookline, Massachusetts, and a lecturer at Harvard Medical School. She is a former Senior Psychiatrist and Director of the Family Therapy Research and Training Program at Judge Baker Guidance Center in Boston, as well as a former consultant in child psychiatry and family therapy at Massachusetts Mental Health Center.

Preface

Other than those who specialize in working with children, most psychotherapists rarely involve children effectively in clinical practice. This is true for family therapists, those who are expected to understand and incorporate in their treatment all members of the system. It is with special joy, then, that the *Journal of Psychotherapy & the Family* is pleased to present this special issue focusing on children in family therapy treating and training.

The purpose of the collection is to provide the practicing psychotherapist with a comprehensive array of well-written, accurate, authoritative, and relevant information vital to working with clients about interpersonal and family-related issues. This volume, with its concern about the integration of child psychology, child psychiatry and a variety of psychotherapy approaches to effectively treating children within the family context, fits this mission extremely well.

One of the most knowledgeable family psychotherapists about children in family therapy is Joan J. Zilbach, MD. Dr. Zilbach recently wrote the highly praised book, *Young Children in Family Therapy* (New York: Brunner/Mazel, 1986). Here she expands on her approach and provides an important historical and conceptual overview soliciting and editing the papers of colleagues working in this important area.

Dr. Zilbach is the former Director of Family Therapy Training Program at the Judge Baker Guidance Center of Boston. Currently she is in independent practice of psychiatry in Boston specializing in the treatment of young children. She is a member of the national training faculty of the Fielding Institute, Santa Barbara, California. Moreover, she gives frequent workshops and presentations on the topic of young children and family therapy and serves in a number of roles in professional organizations and publications. We are very fortunate to have Dr. Zilbach as the editor of this important special collection.

All of the contributors to this collection were carefully selected for the special expertise in the treatment of children within a family

1

context. The collection includes 10 papers divided among two sections dealing with treatment and training. These contributors are well-known and respected psychiatrists, psychologists, social workers, and family therapists who effectively summarize their précis of effectively working with children in family therapy.

As a father of an 11-year old (Jessica) and a 3-year old (Laura) I was impressed with the insight of Dr. Zilbach and her contributors to both the capabilities and limitations of children at various ages. I have not only learned about how to effectively involve a child like Laura in my practice, but also some useful methods in getting through the day as a parent! I am sure that the readers will enjoy this book personally and professionally.

Charles R. Figley, PhD
Editor, Journal of Psychotherapy & the Family

Introduction and Overview

Joan J. Zilbach

Family therapy, a relatively young psychotherapeutic modality, wears like Joseph, a coat of many colors. The general title "Psychotherapy and the Family" reflects the change that occurred in the mid-1950s when the family became a potential unit of treatment in psychotherapy rather than only an individual patient/client. From the beginning of this clinical practice several important theories developed which influenced the emerging schools of family therapy. This special volume, *Children in Family Therapy: Treatment and Training*, is devoted to an aspect of family therapy that has received little attention. The field has developed a practice of including "talking" adult members and excluding non-verbal playing children. The family therapists in this volume with varying theoretical orientations all have one belief and practice in common, that children are integral members of the family as a unit and should not be excluded from the therapeutic arena.

Nowadays in this still rapidly growing field with its ranges of theories and techniques, practitioners when they do meet can easily identify and establish their particular positions within the spectrum of family therapies. They know their own color amongst the many in the family therapy coat! However, representatives of the main schools often present in their own separate places or write their own books. In this volume, treating children in their families has brought family therapy practitioners of various schools together.

HISTORY

The place of children in the history of family therapy is worth noting. There are several versions of the overall historical development of family therapy in the family therapy literature. (See Guerin, 1976; Gurman and Kniskern, 1981; Zilbach, 1986 and others.)

3

However, as a general statement, in the beginning there were two main "branches," "East Coast" and "West Coast," and some other isolated individuals pioneering the early discoveries and practice of family therapy.

East Coast Branch

This branch included as early members Nathan Ackerman, Bowen, Minuchin, Wynne amongst others. One of the earliest books in family therapy was Nathan Ackerman's *The Psychodynamics of Family Life* (1958). Ackerman, a child psychiatrist and psychoanalyst, became a pioneer in family therapy who worked intensively with children in their families. The Ackerman Institute under his influence and others, and also previously as part of the child guidance movement, always included children in their family therapy sessions. Some of Ackerman's early videotapes are still worth studying to learn directly about children in actual family treatment sessions. The East Coast branch with a psychoanalytic theoretical base has continued to flourish, create new branches and promote both the development of theory and many practitioners.

West Coast Branch

The West Coast branch originating at the same time as the East Coast included well-known members such as Bateson, Jackson, Haley, and Satir. These family therapists amongst others with Bateson as a leader, developed their theoretical base from general systems theory and cybernetics, and this has become present-day "family systems" theory (Bateson, 1971). General systems theory to a varying extent has dominated all branches of family therapy (Bertalanffy, 1968, Hoffman, 1981).

Curiously, while a systemic "whole family" orientation has continued as a theoretical base, in practice, non-verbal and non-adult child members began to be eliminated by this school from the therapeutic scene as communications, strategic and other sub-theories began to emerge in practice. Of course, any such generalizations have their exceptions. On the West Coast Virginia Satir published her classic volume *Conjoint Family Therapy* in 1964, and there was a chapter in the first version entitled "Including the Children in Family Therapy" (Satir, 1964). The "strategic" school with J. Haley as its center certainly has always and continues to include young children (Haley, 1973).

Carl Whitaker has his own brand of family therapy which cannot be neatly classified (Whitaker, 1982). He too has always included children and his writings contain some of the most vivid and expressive examples of including children of all ages from babies to adolescents.

PLAY IN FAMILY TREATMENT

When children are included in family sessions their natural language, play, becomes an important part of the family session. Though the orientation of the family therapists may differ, children's play reaches across the spectrum of the schools of both treatment and training in this volume.

"Go away, and play" is a frequent adult dismissal when children are at the least in the way, or annoying and even disruptive of adult conversation. And yet, play is often the expressive and primary basic language of children. This language with its many activities is characteristic of children of all ages and even some adults. Children do not conform to the adult "talking" model of psychotherapy. As exemplified in the treatment examples, they do not sit still, nor do they only play—some even "hurl themselves" as in one of our cases (see in this volume, "Systemic Family Therapy with Young Children and Their Families: Use of the Reflecting Team," Lax). Some adults leave most of their play both in action and language behind as they "mature"! When this occurs in therapists it becomes difficult for them to understand and appreciate what children do in family therapy sessions. It is most important to realize how serious and valuable these play activities are – play is child's work. In order to understand children's play, child training is useful as part of an introduction to the inclusion of children in family therapy, or, at least, to be grounded in child development. However, even without this formal induction children can be included in simple ways in family sessions. In each of the papers there are examples of the inclusion of children, the use of simple toys, and understanding simple productions, drawings, etc. (For further details see the papers and books in the resources section – "Specific References to Children in Family Therapy.")

FAMILY DEVELOPMENT
AND THE FAMILY LIFE CYCLE

Another aspect of the understanding of family therapy held in common by the writers in this volume, to a greater or lesser extent, is the concept of the family life cycle and family development i.e., the family as a whole unit changing in its own particular ways over a course of the span of any one family unit. In recent years increasing attention has been devoted in the family therapy literature to the family life cycle. Family development across the span of the years of the family life cycle is a way of understanding some of the complexities within family therapy (Zilbach, 1979, 1988). Children occupy a particularly prominent position in the early phases of family development.

One model of the family life cycle is discussed in the chapter in this volume "Child and Family Therapy: An Integrated Approach" by Drs. Gordetsky and Zilbach, pp. 95-115 (for others see Combrinck-Graham, 1985; Carter and McGoldrick, 1980).

THE PLAYERS: THE CONTRIBUTORS

All contributors to this collection are seasoned practitioners of family therapy working in a variety of settings, operating from various theoretical vantage points and include children of all ages in their therapeutic endeavors. Their pathways into this work are as diverse as their professional backgrounds and theoretical positions as indicated in their answers to my query, "How did you become interested in treating children in family therapy?" Their fascinating responses deserve to be quoted in full. However, this was not possible and excerpts follow.

Dr. Richard Chasin, Director of the Family Institute of Cambridge, the author of the opening article on "Interviewing Families with Children: Guidelines and Suggestions" had interviewed over 200 families and, "'I thought of myself as a family therapist even though none of the families I had seen included a young child." At that time, 1966, he began training in child psychiatry and subsequently felt comfortable with children and began to include them in family sessions. Later when he was responsible for family therapy teaching, he looked for teaching tapes:

I eagerly sought tapes of masters. . . . I was surprised when I realized how few included children and I was often horrified by those that did. The children were generally treated like a homunculi, shrunken adults, frozen into chairs, trying to cope with language and content that was beyond their developmental reach.

Since that time he has vigorously continued this interest as "a minor crusade to help clinicians deal constructively with children in family therapy."

In the second paper, Dr. Lee Combrinck-Graham utilizes her strong theoretical family systems approach to understand borderline syndrome in childhood. About the origins of her interest:

Many child/family therapists added the family to their child work. I began with the child in the family . . . trained at the Philadelphia Child Guidance Clinic where children were always seen in families, despite the general disapproval of Philadelphia's child psychiatry community.

Her child/family orientation has remained steady throughout the years in varying mental health contexts. In her present position as Director of the Institute for Juvenile Research, and Director of the Division of Child and Adolescent Psychiatry at the University of Illinois, she puts an emphasis on poor children, ". . . where children are undereducated . . . have little motivation to push for success in a society that offers few rewards to them." This work promises an expansion of our understanding of children in families — in poor families.

The title of the third paper, "Systemic Family Therapy with Young Children and Their Families: Use of the Reflecting Team," adds the next theoretical orientation. Dr. Lax, presently the Director of the Brattleboro Family Institute, was trained as a Gestalt therapist. He attributes his present orientation to his work in the past few years with Lynn Hoffman, "I was originally trained as a Gestalt therapist, taught to be respectful of individuals' organic processes in therapy." After becoming involved in family therapy, he looked for a model that contained some of the values that I had found in Gestalt therapy: respect for the client; not being an expert who always knew what was "best" for the client; not being "responsible" for change; and attending to what was the "presenting edge" of treatment. . . . Lynn (Hoffman) taught me how to think theoretically and to question. . . . Four years ago (I was) introduced . . . to Tom Anderson and his "reflecting team" model. It was a "difference that made a difference." . . . The model is always developing, without any fixed ideas of "how it should be done." I still feel like an adventurer, never getting there, but always arriving.

Dr. David E. Scharff, the author of the fourth paper, "Young Children and Play in Object Relations Family Therapy," presently Director of The Washington School of Psychiatry, attributes his interest to

my first long-term family case . . . as a resident. There the youngest child, a six year old, drew and the latency children commented on his drawings. It was obvious there was more life in the children's play than in the more sedate words of the adults.

His theoretical interest in object relations deepened and has been integrated into his family work:

The non-verbal contributions even of the infants in a family had an important organizing influence on the family even as the family "organized" the infant. The mutuality of these interactions between adults and young children could only be understood — as any child therapist knows — by the use of play and the observation of non-verbal and pre-verbal information. . . . Of course, even with all this rationale, there is also the fact that it's more fun to have the young children there and that their forthrightness is generally refreshing.

Next, Dr. Scholfield-MacNab, Boston Institute of Psychotherapies, explores in depth one aspect of object relations family therapy i.e., countertransference in family therapy with children. Her interest in working with children began with an early training experience on an inpatient adolescent unit:

> I co-led one of the first family groups in this very psychodynamic, individually-oriented hospital, and became intrigued with the possibilities for change within families, not just individuals. It was also a great relief to move outside of the "blaming the parents" stance that seemed so prevalent.

She continued her family work in a community mental health clinic and private practice retaining

> an enthusiasm for family therapy . . . with its premise of treating the context of the identified patient's problem, their family. . . . (It is) effective, more humane . . . not asking the child to be "disloyal" by changing when his family was not involved with change . . . , and more exciting . . . to see the often startling impact of systemic interactions and interventions.

The last paper in the Treatment section, "Child and Family Therapy: An Integrated Approach" co-authored by Dr. Gordetsky, Chief Psychologist, Parents' and Children's Services (Boston) and myself, is the product of many years of joint family therapy endeavors. Dr. Gordetsky's interest began

> As a graduate student in child development and clinical psychology I elected to join a family therapy seminar offered at the Judge Baker Guidance Center where I was (previously) learning (only) individual and group child therapy.

This seminar was part of the program my colleagues and I developed at the Judge Baker Guidance Center. The fun, freshness and liveliness that children bring to family sessions have been noted by previous contributors. Dr. Gordetsky includes the other side — pain and poignancy, ". . . In the beginning family sessions were sometimes difficult; but they were also poignant and touching. Family sessions appeared to help all members of the family and to prevent potential future problems. The effort seemed worth it."

The first paper in the Training section is a comprehensive presentation of training at the Jewish Board of Family and Children's Services in New York City. The senior author, Dr. Clifford J. Sager, Director of Family Psychiatry and Codirector Advanced Training Programs, Jewish Board of Family and Children's Services, New York City, had an early start in "family sessions":

> As a boiling-over nine year old in [my] "latency" period, [I] became the patient. [Dr. T.] would often spend part of a session with my mother, occasionally with my father and sometimes with both me and my parents. . . . Early on I concluded that the Oedipus complex was only one narrow aspect of family dynamics. I learned that children and adults reacted very differently when together with different combinations of family members. This prompted me to decide to see both marital partners together. With this format I could immediately witness regressive behavior and transferential reactions that spouses had to each other. Shortly after that I began to include children with their parents in evaluation sessions insisting that babes-in-arms be brought in too. . . . In 1964 Nat Ackerman's generosity in inviting my staff and me to his weekly one-way mirror family sessions at Jewish Family Service moved me into family therapy . . .

His co-author and colleague at Jewish Board of Family Children's Services, Connie Moss-Kagel, states directly:

> I, Connie Moss-Kagel, work with young children in family therapy as a result of both personal and professional influences. Being a middle child in a sibship of eight children, I strove for individuation and autonomy in a complex family with powerful pulls . . . the dialectic between the individual and the family have been charged areas of interest for me . . . early childcare tasks established the conditions under which responsibilities were discharged while playing, a combination appreciated by my charges. The establishment of my own family with my husband, Murray, and the pleasure of raising my daughter, Nicole, allowed me to explore from the parental position the issues of the individual and the family . . .

Dr. Abramovitz is Chief of Psychiatry and Codirector of the Advanced Training Program in Child and Family Treatment at the Jewish Family and Children's Services. After training at the Yale Child Study Center his work in a health center with a low income population precipitated him into family work: "There was no way to see these children without their families. Lots of kids were referred and everybody in the family warred with each other rather than contending with what they had to . . ."

In the next paper on training, my co-author, Dr. Michael I. Bennett, Director of Adult Outpatient Services, Massachusetts Mental Health Center, states boldly:

> I became interested in including children in family work at the time I began my own family . . . This experience made me comfortable with the child's ability to destroy a parent's composure in a family interview. . . . (I could) enjoy the process of continuing the (family) interview and learning about family interactions as they really occurred.

Family experiences in the therapist's own and others, including patient families, are the foundation of the training seminar described in this paper.

Play, as an important part of training for family therapists, is the topic of Dr. Jill Savege Scharff's paper. She is presently Coordinator of the Psychoanalytic Family Therapy Training Program, Child Section of the Washington School of Psychiatry and has had training in child and adult psychoanalysis, and community psychiatry. Her experience in emergency room consultation with family interviewing was a formative influence,

> Access to the family system could readily be obtained during crisis and this paved the way for a family therapy approach. . . . Raising (my) own family of young children while dealing with stepchildren through their adolescence was another impetus to regarding the whole family as a unit of interest.

The last paper adds some research validation to our treatment and training endeavors. Jeannette R. Kramer, Staff and Faculty of the Center for Family Studies/The Family Institute of Chicago, states:

> I cannot even think about transgenerational issues without thinking of the newest members — the children — and how they will be impacted by, and make an impact on the family . . . I have lived and worked with the transgenerational spectrum. In my first career (1946-1956) my primary focus was launching 6 children born to my husband Chuck and myself . . . I have always been curious about changes and how what is learned in one context can be passed on to another . . . the natural progression to transfer learning. I believe that changes within family of origin members are basic and likely to transfer most easily to other interfaces.

In this paper the "transfer" to the children of therapists in her training groups and the validation of the effects by the questionnaires, broadens and intensifies our view of training and the "transfer" or effects of family of origin work on children.

Finally, as the editor of this collection and also a contributor, a co-author, to both the Treatment and Training sections, I asked myself the same question about how my interest in including children in family therapy developed. I became part of the "East Coast Branch" in the mid-1950s when immediately after my training in child psychiatry on my first job as a staff member on a research project I was plunged into families by the delinquent girls in a research project. These girls did not understand the "individuals only" rules of the treatment game and spontaneously included their family members. Since the field was just beginning, there was no training at that time and fortunately I attended a family meeting at the American Orthopsychiatric Association where I met embryonic family therapists (Minuchin, Auerswald, Wynne and others) who were puzzling about family therapeutic issues. Shortly thereafter, I and a small group of colleagues began a "pilot project" on treating families. This interest has continued up to the present. The early period of treating families also coincided with the beginning and growth of my own family which was very productive! As I continued my work in family treatment I also became a psychoanalyst. My present theoretical interest in the family life cycle and family development is a combination of my past in child development, psychoanalysis, my own family and a continuing interest in family theory. However, my own family and family of origin have taught me the most and sustained and supported me/us through our family lives together.

As noted in the authors' biographical comments, this collection of articles includes a range of backgrounds and theoretical orientations which influence training and treatment of children in family therapy. The intent of this work is to encourage other family therapists to consider treating the whole family, including its younger members who will become the parents of the next generation of children.

ACKNOWLEDGMENTS

My first to my husband and family for patience, support, creative inquiry and family ideas. Professionally I have had two co-teachers at the Fielding Institute, Dr. Clinton Phillips and Dr. Suzanne Jensen. In addition, the many students and families particularly their children have been invaluable contributors in family learning. And last, the authors of this volume have been generous in their contributions. Thank you.

REFERENCES

Ackerman, N.W. (1958). *The psychodynamics of family life*. New York: Basic Books.
Bateson, G. (1971). *Steps to an ecology of mind*. New York: Ballantine Books.
Bertalanffy, von. L.V. (1968). *General systems theory*. New York: Braziller.
Bowen, M. (1978). *Family therapy in clinical practice*. New York: Jason Aronson.
Carter, E., & McGoldrick, M. (Eds.) (1980). *The family life cycle: A framework for family therapy*. New York: Gardner Press.
Combrinck-Graham, L. (1985). A developmental model for family systems. *Family Process, 24*, 139-151.
Guerin, P.J. (Ed.) (1976). *Family therapy: Theory and practice*. New York: Gardner Press.
Gurman, A.S., & Kniskern, D.P. (1981b). *Handbook of family therapy*. New York: Brunner/Mazel.
Haley, J. (1973). Strategic therapy when a child is presented as a problem. *Journal of the American Academy of Child Psychiatry, 12*, 641-659.
Hoffman, L. (1981). *Foundations of family therapy*. New York: Basic Books.

Jackson, D.D. (1957). The question of family homeostasis. *Psychiatry Quarterly Supplement, 31*, 79-90. Reprinted in: *International Journal of Family Therapy*, 1981, 3(1), 5-16.

Minuchin, S. (1974). *Families and family therapy*. Cambridge, MA: Harvard University Press.

Sager, C.J., & Kaplan, H.S. (1972). *Progress in group and family therapy*. New York: Brunner/Mazel.

Satir, V.W. (1964). *Conjoint family therapy*. Palo Alto: Science & Behavior Books.

Scharff, D., & Scharff, J. (1987). *Object relations family therapy*. Northvale, NJ: Jason Aronson, Inc.

Weakland, J. (1960). The double-bind hypothesis of schizophrenia and three party interaction. In D.D. Jackson (Ed.), *The etiology of schizophrenia* (p. 374). New York: Basic Books.

Whitaker, C. (1982). *From psyche to system: The evolving therapy of Carl Whitaker*. J.R. Neill & D.P. Kniskern (Eds.). New York: Guilford Press.

Wynne, L. (1965). Some indications and contraindications for exploratory family therapy. In I. Boszormenyi-Nagy, & J.L. Framo (Eds.), *Intensive family therapy* (pp. 289-322). New York: Harper & Row.

Zilbach, J.J. (1968). Family development. In J. Marmor (Ed.), *Modern psychoanalysis* (pp. 355-386). New York: Basic Books.

Zilbach, J.J. (1979). Family development and familial factors in etiology. In J. Noshpitz et al. (Eds.), *Basic handbook of child psychiatry*, Vol. II (pp. 62-87). New York: Basic Books.

Zilbach, J.J. (1982). Separation: A family developmental process of midlife years. In C. Nadelson & M. Notman (Eds.), *The woman patient*, Vol. II (pp. 159-167). New York: Plenum Press.

Zilbach, J.J. (1988). The family life cycle: A framework for understanding children in family therapy. In L. Combrinck-Graham (Ed.), *Children in Family Contexts* (pp. 46-66). New York: Guilford Press.

Interviewing Families with Children: Guidelines and Suggestions

Richard Chasin

INTRODUCTION

One of the great common failings in the current practice of child therapy and of family therapy is that in neither case is there sufficient use of whole family sessions including children. Child therapists tend to interview children without adults present and family therapists often leave out children, especially young ones. A major reason for these exclusions is that little effort has been made to develop the techniques necessary for conducting joint sessions.

Numerous authors have sung the praises of whole family sessions for enriching the therapist's understanding of both child and family, and also as a setting in which intervention can be particularly effective (Ackerman, 1966; Zilbach, Bergel & Gass; 1972; Bloch, 1976). But the literature is relatively scant on the subject of techniques which might be useful when the therapist simultaneously interviews family members at different levels of development

Richard Chasin, MD, is Director of the Family (Therapy) Institute of Cambridge, Watertown, MA and Associate Clinical Professor of Psychiatry at Cambridge Hospital, Harvard Medical School, Cambridge, MA.

15

(Villeneuve, 1979; Keith, 1986; Zilbach, 1986, Chasen & White, 1989).

In this paper I shall outline briefly some considerations about the use of play and about the office set-up, and then offer general guidelines and specific suggestions to help therapists keep children in their families during assessment and treatment sessions.

PLAY AND PLAYTHINGS

Any interviewer who wishes to fully engage young children should be prepared to use play as a medium of communication. Play does not necessarily involve toys. In fact, no equipment is required for role-playing, which is the most flexible, revealing and impactful play technique in the therapist's treasure chest. When toys are made available they should be ones that an adult can comfortably use and should lend themselves to play which is easy to interpret. It may be fun for a three-year old to spill marbles over the floor and kick them around, but the grown-ups will probably not join in or learn much from the child's preference for dispersing the red ones rather than the green ones. By contrast, hand-puppets, dolls, and crayon drawings foster play that is more intelligible and collaborative for people of all ages.

In family sessions, the therapist will usually be more directive than in individual play therapy sessions. He or she will often have to decide when to play, what to play, how to play, who joins in, and who watches. Even with these decisions in the therapist's hands there will be plenty of room for spontaneity. If the therapist is too non-directive, impulsive families will become chaotic and repressed ones will freeze in the face of so much freedom.

THE INTERVIEWING ROOM

Offices that are specifically set up either for adults or for children are not necessarily good spaces in which to conduct whole family interviews. Spaces designed for grown-ups will not be sufficiently child-proofed and the child may feel alienated by the formal furnishings and lack of toys. The parents and therapist will be nervous about elaborate equipment or delicate art objects that may be within the reach of naturally curious children. Settings which are suitable for children often feel uncomfortable to adults, who may be cramped in small chairs and menaced by the presence of paints and clay that could soil the fine clothing they have worn to impress the therapist.

The best workspace is relatively bare, and contains only moveable chairs and a few cushions. Initially, most of the toys and equipment should be kept in cabinets and drawers. The therapist decides which ones to bring into the room, and when. I have described elsewhere an ideal arrangement of space and facilities which allows observation from behind a one-way mirror, has a time-out space, and provides play and talk areas which may be joined together or separated from each other (Chasin, 1981).

THE EVALUATION PROCESS

When a family is being assessed, a child is usually the index case. In such instances, the least complicated way to proceed is for the therapist first to interview the parents and/or other caretakers in order to get oriented and to gather information about the membership and workings of the household, the development of the children, the families of origin, the relationship among the adults responsible for day-to-day care, the context in which the present problems arose and the solutions which have been attempted. Some of this data is best discussed without the children present. It is prudent to spare children the tedium of insurance data or the burden of learning details of their parents' sexual life. However, any information gathered in the parent session which is appropriate and interesting for children can be addressed again when the whole family meets together.

Many family therapists prefer to see the whole family together first, with no prior parental interview. While such an approach has the advantages of fostering an unbiased stance and a clear focus on the family unit, it can be risky, especially for a therapist inexperienced in either family or child work. The therapist may feel forced to choose between attending to the children while ignoring the adults, or getting complex background information from the adults, thus provoking disruptive behavior from the children. By contrast, the therapist who interviews the parents first has already gathered considerable information and begun to join with them. This therapist can afford to concentrate more on the children in the full family session, because the parents will not feel neglected. He or she will also be prepared by the parent session for some of the special problems and opportunities that will present themselves when the whole family is interviewed.

The following procedure is useful for whole family sessions during the assessment process (Chasin, Roth & Bograd, 1989). Some of these suggestions will be irrelevant or inadequate for specific cases. However, the recommended steps can serve as a guide, especially for those readers who have not yet developed an approach of their own.

Step 1: The Therapist Explains the Reason for the Family Meeting

I have seen experienced therapists begin interviews by asking the children, "What did your parents tell you this meeting was about?" or "Why do you think we are here?" Frequently parents have not prepared children for the meeting and sometimes they have even lied to them about it. In those cases, the session gets off to an awkward start with the parents confronted by their incompetence or dishonesty.

It is better for the therapist to begin the session by introducing himself or herself and asking the family members how they would like to be addressed. Once introductions are over, the therapist takes responsibility for the session by immediately telling the family members why he or she has assembled everyone and what it is that they can expect. This requires the therapist to disclose the gist of prior contacts with the parents and other informants and to indicate the purpose of the whole family session.

In this opening step, the content that is shared and the simple phrasing that is used by the therapist should model respectful candor and reflect the therapist's wish that all members of the family understand and participate in the meeting. A conscious effort should be made throughout the sessions to ensure that the language and sentence structure used is easily comprehended by children and adults and that each member of the group is treated with equal respect.

> *Therapist (to each parent and then to each child)*: What name would you like me to call you?

> *Family members reply*: (Mother is Ellen. Father, Dan. Children, Eric, seven and Susie, five)

> *Therapist (to everyone)*: My name is Dr. Chasin. You may call me Dick if you would like to. My work is to help families find ways to make things better for themselves when everything is not all right. Ellen and Dan called me on the phone the other day and told me that you have a good family but that everyone in the family was unhappy in some way. They said Susie has been sad and has scary dreams. They told me that her teacher says she is unhappy in school, too. When I heard all that, I asked Dan and Ellen to visit me here in this room.

> *Therapist (continuing)*: We met a few days ago and talked about Susie. They said they were also a little worried about Eric who seems angry a lot. They even said they themselves disagreed a lot with each other and fought sometimes. After we talked I told them that I would like to meet with everyone in the family. What we are going to do here today is to talk and play so that you can find new ways for the family to be happier.

Step 2: Therapist Sets the Rules for the Meeting

It can be terrifying for anyone to play a game without knowing the rules, particularly if the stakes are high. Yet many therapists will conduct family meetings without having established even the most rudimentary contract. Whether or not a contract has been made in a prior parent session (and I would hope it has), the therapist should explicitly set out rules for the whole family interview. At the minimum, it is wise to make agreements about non-coercion, safety, discipline, and use of the space and equipment.

Therapist (to everyone): Before we begin I want to tell you the rules. First, you should not answer a question or do anything I ask unless you feel ready to do it. If you do not feel ready to answer a question or do something I ask, just don't do it and it will be all right. If you wish, you can tell me that you are not ready by saying the word "pass" or "not now" or something like that.

The second rule is that Dan and Ellen are responsible for discipline. If Eric or Susie does something that is not allowed at home, then Ellen and Dan should do here just what they would do at home.

The third rule is that we all try to make sure that everyone is safe. If somebody does something that might cause a cut or a bruise, everyone here should help to stop it from happening.

The last rule is that I decide what toys we use and when we use them.

After the rules are stated, the therapist makes sure they are understood and are agreed on by everyone. In some cases, the therapist may need to make agreements about other matters, such as confidentiality and videotaping. It is indeed a challenge to establish boundaries and define expectations briefly enough not to exhaust the patience of the family but clearly enough so that the rules are understood by everyone who can possibly comprehend them.

Without rules the family may experience iatrogenic anxiety and their behavior can be misleading. I have seen children so badgered by a parent to "answer the doctor's question" that the doctor regrets ever having asked it. With the non-coercion or "pass" rule in place, the therapist can say, "Your son has just passed. Thank you for trying to help me but it is my problem, not yours. I need to think of questions he is ready to answer."

Step 3: Joining

After the rules are established, the therapist can begin to interact more extensively with the family. The word "joining" rather than "alliance building" has been used by family therapists for this early period of exchange because the therapist does not simply ally, but temporarily becomes part of the family or, more precisely, becomes a member of a new system, the therapist-family system. While many therapists tailor their joining methods to each individual family, I almost always join by asking family members to tell me their strengths. By always using the same approach, I learn a great deal from families right away because I have a yardstick of extensive comparable experience to apply. Furthermore, this method is almost always agreeable to families, and it starts the session off on a distinctly positive note.

> *Therapist (to everyone)*: If I am going to help you find a way to figure out how to make things better, I first need to know what power, strength and ability you all have. I'll ask each of you to tell us about something that you are good at doing, something that you know how to do and are proud about. I'd like to start with Eric.
>
> *Eric*: I have good friends.
>
> *Therapist*: What is it about you that makes it possible for you to have good friends?
>
> *Eric*: Kids like me. I don't tell them lies and junk.

The father might mention that he works hard and supports his family no matter what. Mother might indicate that she too is a hard worker and that she protects her children. The daughter might say she is nice, that she is no trouble to anyone.

The therapist continues until each of the family members has described two or three positive character elements. Young children often interpret this inquiry as referring to things they like, rather than to abilities. However, for anything a child likes, the therapist can suggest a skill that such a preference reflects. When this mode of joining is used, the family is relieved that the therapist is not dragging out the worst problems immediately. Indeed, the family's morale is strengthened by discussing its strengths. In multi-problem families with poor self-esteem, the members may expect disrespectful treatment from therapists. They are sometimes deeply moved when a therapist is interested in celebrating their strengths.

Step 4: Exploration of the Family's Goals and Problems

No aspect of an evaluation interview is more important than the manner of the therapist's exploration of goals and problems. Each school of therapy, indeed each clinician, charts a different course and employs a different style for this investigation. My own approach is eclectic, borrowing ideas and techniques from various methods to achieve results basic to a good assessment: a therapist with sound information upon which to base recommendations and family members who have not only learned something from the evaluation process, but who also feel good enough about it that they would accept a recommendation for therapy if it were offered.

In the first family interview, it is generally wise and efficient for the therapist to focus on the family's goals and problems and their obviously relevant contexts. Frequently, the resolution of the current difficulty does not require a broad and deep exploration of the remote past or of larger systems, such as the extended family and service agencies. If an initial parent meeting is held, then the therapist can usually decide which, if any, past event or larger systems need to be addressed, and/or represented, in the first whole family session.

The goal and problem exploration phase of the family interview will ordinarily concentrate on problematic behavior patterns and the belief systems which support them, including family ideas about the meaning of the problem and the way it should be solved. It will also be useful to understand the family's hope for the future and their fears about what might happen if the problem were to remain uncorrected.

Obviously, there are many ways to accomplish these ends. The approach I outline here is sufficiently idiosyncratic that I anticipate few will simply adopt it. However, the reader may want to re-consider, and perhaps modify or augment his or her usual methods in the light of the following suggestions.

Hopes

I prefer to start the family session with each person expressing his or her hopes for the future. By delaying the subject of problems, the therapist reduces defensiveness and gives family members greater freedom to show what they are like.

> *Therapist*: I'd like now to give you each a chance to say one or two ways that your family can be better than it already is.

Children's answers are sometimes quite egocentric and concrete. A child may say that things would be better if she had a new toy. It is important that the therapist accept any answer and develop it a bit. "What will this new toy be?" "Who should give it to you?" "Can you draw a picture of it?" By contrast, older children and parents are sometimes quite abstract and negative.

> *Mother*: Eric needs to stop being so rivalrous with his sister.

> *Therapist*: What one thing do you want him to stop?

> *Mother*: Hitting her.

> *Therapist*: If he were to stop hitting, what would you like him to do with her instead?

> *Mother*: I would like him to build things together with her, using her blocks.

After developing a list of hopes, the family should be liberated from words and encouraged to play-out some of these wishes. The therapist can suggest that the family illustrate what might happen if all their dreams were to come true. Ideally, the family members, working collaboratively, create and role-play a scene which weaves these wishes together. Families that are intimidated by this task may follow the therapist's suggestions about how to enact such a skit. Alternatively, the family members, together or separately, can draw a picture showing an ideal future. The point is to engage the family in a joint activity which reflects their hopes for themselves.

Even though the content may be all about an ideal future, the interaction among the family members will reveal to the therapist a great deal about problematic behavior patterns which can be interpreted in whatever way the therapist customarily processes such data. At this point, the therapist should say little, if anything, about provisional hypotheses.

Future Dreads and Current Problems

In some cases, one can continue to postpone the discussion and demonstration of current problems by asking the family to state, and at times illustrate with play, what they are afraid will happen if things continue as they are. This step is particularly helpful when families dispute the details of the problem. It is harder to fight over the correctness of one another's fears than it is to squabble about the accuracy of each other's description of a past event (Lee, 1986).

By this time, the therapist will have learned enough to have some ideas about the nature of the current problem, and the atmosphere in the interview will be positive enough for the family directly to address these present difficulties with relative comfort. Whatever is still unclear to the therapist should determine the continuing approach to this investigation.

If the behavioral sequences that include the problem are fuzzy, the therapist might ask the family member what happens before and after "Susie gets sad" or "Eric becomes angry." Better still, each member, using hand-puppets, can be given a chance to illustrate the sequence of events.

> *Therapist (pointing)*: This puppet is mother, this one is father, that one is Susie, and this other one is Eric. Who would like to show us what happens before mother and father fight?
>
> *Susie*: (volunteers, and picks up the mother and father puppets)
>
> *Susie (as mother)*: Go put Eric to bed.
>
> *Susie (as father)*: Get me a drink.
>
> *Susie (as mother)*: I will not.
>
> *Susie (as father)*: I'm leaving.
>
> *Therapist*: You have shown us a little about what happens before and during a fight. Can you show us what happens afterward?
>
> *Susie*: I won't.

Therapist: Good, You just "passed." Would anyone else like a turn?

Note: when the family demonstrates its painful sequences, it is less of a strain for them to use hand-puppets or dolls than for them to role-play themselves at their worst.

When belief systems rather than behavioral sequences are what the therapist needs to understand further, somewhat different modes of questioning and play are likely to be more successful. Given this end, no method of verbal inquiry is more useful for working with children than some form of the circular, triadic and reflexive questioning developed by systemic therapists of the Milan tradition (Tomm, 1987). For example, the rich tapestry of family beliefs can be unfolded by using simple comparison questions, such as: "Who is the most worried about Susie's sadness?" "Who is the least worried?" "Who is the most annoyed by Eric's anger?" "Who is next most angry?" Children as young as four or five may not only be able to understand and answer such questions, but they often can keep the answers well in mind and learn something from them about the pattern of family beliefs and relationships. Thus they can become informed, active participants in the family's creation of new ways of thinking about themselves and new solutions for their problems.

While many modes of play reveal the belief structures in the family, drawings are especially useful because they contain numerous clues to perceptions and ideas. Children are often not conscious of what they express in drawings. The observer may see more than the artist. The therapist should probably start with specific drawing tasks, such as in the Kinetic Family Drawing (Burns & Kaufman, 1972), where the family members are asked to each make a drawing of the family doing something. The therapist may be more specific and ask for drawings about problematic behavior. However, undirected free drawings (Zilbach, 1986) may also be useful, especially since they are performed in the context of a family meeting and may well give clues to the child's perception of the subjects under discussion.

Mother: Look at Susie's picture. I am so small and colorless. Eric is huge and my husband is colorful. I have always been afraid that I have little influence upon Susie.

Therapist (to father): Who do you think is least important to Susie?

Father: I always thought it was me, but I now see how Ellen could think it was her.

Therapist (to Eric): Your mother and father each thought they were least important to Susie. What do you think?

Eric: Susie doesn't care about me.

Susie: Mommy is very important to me, but she is so quiet.

Mother (to therapist): I didn't tell you this when we met before, but I have been very slowed down since we moved. Dan's drinking doesn't help.

Therapist (to everyone): Who was most upset about the move?

Thus, through play and simple inquiry the family and the therapist can learn about family relationships and their connection with the current problems.

Step 5: The Therapist Gives Impressions and Recommendations

At the end of the whole family interview process, which may take one to three separate sessions, the family members should learn what the therapist thinks of them and what to do next. Such a statement should not be put together hastily. It is often useful to take time out before making it. Some family therapists work with a co-therapist or even a team who brainstorm together—apart from the family—before announcing the clinical impressions and recommendations.

In this closing statement the therapist should refer to the strengths in the family and indicate how, without bad intentions, family members may have developed a pattern of behavior that falls short of their hopes. A clear recommendation should follow.

Therapist: You have a strong and close family. You were mostly happy until the move. Ellen (mother) misses her friends and wants more help than ever from Dan (father). He already had plenty to do in his difficult job and is trying to find some way to calm down, whether it is by drinking or going out with his new friends. Both Dan and Ellen seem to want more from each other than they think they can give. Susie misses the old neighborhood and is sad that her parents are having a hard time. She does not want to add to their troubles, so she is quiet about her sadness and asks for very little. Eric is angry and says things that are painful but true so that the family will do something about its unhappiness.

Therapist (concluding): Now that I know you better, I think you will solve your problems more quickly if we have about six sessions. We can have more meetings than that if it turns out that you are not getting what you hope for when the six sessions are over.

A FEW WORDS ABOUT TREATMENT

Treatment sessions including children require an artful balance of planning and spontaneity. The therapist should determine the general strategy for each session and decide which family members should attend. Sometimes the therapist may want to interview the children without the parents present in order to directly intervene in the sibling relationship without the impediment of the force field created by the adults. Such sibling interviews are of particular importance when the children are the object of parental neglect or when they compete with rather than support one another.

In general, when therapy sessions include children, the clinician should continue to ensure their active involvement no matter what theory guides the treatment. Many schools of family therapy — behavioral, experiential, child-oriented psychodynamic, systemic, structural — have traditions of active engagement of children (Ackerman, 1966; Minuchin, 1974; Forehand, 1977; Palazzoli, Boscolo, Cecchin & Prata, 1978; Neill & Kniskern, 1982) but some — Bowenian and psychodynamic family of origin oriented — do not

(Framo, 1976; Bowen, 1978). It hardly matters. Even schools that have a history of including children may not employ a wide range of techniques. The creative therapist who wishes to work simultaneously with children and adults can invent fresh ways of talking and playing that will serve almost any therapeutic purpose guided by almost any general theory.

When treatment is focussed on the here and now of family life, the therapist can use methods similar to those mentioned in the section on assessment. However, it is often necessary to widen the scope and look at the past and at larger systems. This can be accomplished in two ways. First, representatives of the families of origin and involved agencies may be included in the sessions. Second, the subject of the sessions can be past occurrences and larger systems. Of course, both devices may be used simultaneously.

After remarriage, blended families often have problems of structure and loyalties. Even if ex-spouses are not available, the whole newly blended group can usefully perform a series of scenes representing a succession of stages starting from the original families and ending with the current situation. By acting out a simple tableau that illustrates the home setting and the relationships at each stage, the whole family becomes mindful of lingering loyalties and old structures that need to be noticed and honored before any new blended family image can be established.

More extensive reenactments of the past may be useful when one child is scapegoated because of projections originating in images from one or both families of origin. Years ago, I worked with a case in which there were strong mythic figures of good and evil in the remote past of father's family. The nine-year-old boy in the current family, a sluggish school failure, had been unaccountably shunned by his father since the day he was born. The family reenacted myth-like events drawn from the lore of father's family. In each of these events the despised child played the hero while the other family members rotated through the evil roles. These enactments confused the family belief system about good and evil and created new images of the rejected child. Subsequently, the child's relationship with his father improved and, after further similar interventions, he became more active and productive.

In another case, both latency children in a family derided their father for his sad sack attitude and his slavish devotion to his own demanding parents whom the children intensely resented. When father reenacted scenes from his childhood, his children could see the degree of his own parents' sacrifice for him. Along the lines of a contextual approach (Boszormenyi-Nagy & Spark, 1973), the children decided that they could be nicer to their grandparents, liberating the father to pay more attention to his children and himself.

CONCLUSION

The challenge for family and child therapists in conducting whole family sessions is to discover how to simultaneously involve family members who are at different levels of development. Whatever the therapist's favored viewpoint or style, children can almost always be profitably included. The guidelines and specific suggestions in this paper are offered as tools for the use of child and family therapists who wish to modify and augment their usual practices to achieve more and better conjoint engagement of both children and adults in evaluation and treatment.

REFERENCES

Ackerman, N. W. (1966). *Treating the troubled family*. New York: Basic Books.
Bloch, D. A. (1976). Are young children necessary in family therapy? In P. Guerin (Ed.), *Family therapy* (pp. 168-181). New York: Gardner Press.
Bowen, M. (1978). *Family therapy in clinical practice*. New York: Jason Aronson.
Boszormenyi-Nagy, I. & Spark, G. M. (1973). *Invisible loyalties: Reciprocity in intergenerational family therapy*. New York: Harper & Row.
Burns, R. C. & Kaufman, S. H. (1972). *Actions, styles and symbols in Kinetic Family Drawings (K-F-D)*. New York: Brunner/Mazel.
Chasin, R. (1981). Involving latency and preschool children in family therapy. In A. Gurman (Ed.), *Questions and answers in the practice of family therapy* (pp. 32-35). New York: Brunner/Mazel.
Chasin, R., Roth, S., & Bograd, M. (1989). Action methods in systemic therapy: Dramatizing ideal futures and reformed pasts with couples. *Family Process*, in press.
Chasin, R. & White, T. (1989). The child in family therapy: Guidelines for active engagement across the age span. In L. Combrinck-Graham (Ed.), *Children in Family Contexts* (pp. 5-25). New York: Guilford Press.
Forehand, R. (1977). Child non-compliance to parental requests: Behavioral anal-

ysis and treatment. In M. Hersen, R. M. Eisler & P. M. Miller (Eds.), *Progress in behavior modification* (vol. 5, pp. 111-143). New York: Academic Press.

Framo, J. L. (1976). Family of origin as a therapeutic resource for adults in marital and family therapy: You can and should go home again. *Family Process*, 15, 193-210.

Keith, D. V. (1986). Are children necessary in family therapy? In L. Combrinck-Graham (Ed.), *Treating young children in family therapy* (pp. 1-10). Rockville, MD: Aspen Publishers, Inc.

Lee, R. (1986). The family therapy trainer as coaching double. *Journal of Group Psychotherapy, Psychodrama and Sociometry*, 39 (2), 52-57.

Minuchin, S. (1974). *Families and family therapy*. Cambridge, MA: Harvard University Press.

Neill, J. R. & Kniskern, D. P. (1982). *From psyche to system: The evolving therapy of Carl Whitaker*. New York: Guilford Press.

Palazzoli, M. S., Boscolo, L., Cecchin, S., & Prata, G. (1978). *Paradox and counterparadox*. New York: Jason Aronson.

Tomm, K. M. (1987). Interventive interviewing: Part II. Reflexive questioning as a means to enable self-healing. *Family Process*, 26 (2), 167-183.

Villeneuve, C. (1979). The specific participation of the child in family therapy. *Journal of the American Academy of Child Psychiatry*, 18 (1), 44-53.

Zilbach, J. J. (1986). *Young children in family therapy*. New York: Brunner/Mazel.

Zilbach, J. J., Bergel, E., & Gass, C. (1972). Role of the young child in family therapy. In C. J. Sager & H. S. Kaplan (Eds.), *Progress in group and family therapy* (pp. 385-399). New York: Brunner/Mazel.

The Borderline Syndrome in Childhood: A Family Systems Approach

Lee Combrinck-Graham

INTRODUCTION

The borderline syndrome and its more established relative, Borderline Personality Disorder, have troubled diagnosticians and nosologists since the idea of a borderline classification emerged in the 1950s (Shapiro, 1983). Originally the category was to cover a large population of puzzling patients who appeared to be neither psychotic nor neurotic. But as interest in characterizing this class of patients grew there was more emphasis on the psychic structure and dynamics of individuals classified as borderline. Thus, while originally "borderline" meant literally on the border between clearer regions of nosology and descriptive phenomenology, today it more fully represents a psychodynamically hypothesized structure which explains the phenomena of impulsivity, affective storms, and fluctuating emotional states.

Family systems theory focuses on the contextual aspects of behavior rather than the intrapsychic aspects. Thus it is difficult for the family therapist to think in terms of borderline phenomena as they have come to be described in contemporary literature. When the family systems oriented therapist considers treatment of what others refer to as the borderline child, it is necessary to reassess the child in terms of his family context rather than in terms of his intra-

Lee Combrinck-Graham, MD, is Director, Institute for Juvenile Research and Director, Division of Child and Adolescent Psychiatry, University of Illinois Medical School.

A version of this paper was presented at Abbott Northwestern Symposium on the Borderline Child in March 1986.

31

psychic life. This reassessment is not simply a translation of terms, but is based on a different way of understanding human behavior.

LANGUAGE, SYNTAX, EPISTEMOLOGY, AND UNDERSTANDING BEHAVIOR

What, besides accent, distinguishes a foreigner speaking English from a native English speaker? Beyond details of idiom, it is grammar and syntax that gives away the foreigner. The native German speaker, for example, constructs sentences the verbs at the end usually putting. This kind of structure actually influences the way some think. The Contextual school, an important family therapy approach developed by Ivan Boszormeny-Nagy, has at its foundations, concepts of trust and loyalty. Nagy observes that these concepts are well understood in countries with a Germanic base to the language, such as Holland, Germany, and Switzerland, while it has been slow to catch on in countries where romance languages are spoken. These important words have quite different meanings in French, Spanish, and Italian than they do in English, Dutch, and German.

In contemplating linguistic differences as wide as Hopi and English, as spoken by Aristotelian Americans, Dell (1980a) observed that the differing world views shaped by the languages could result in major misunderstandings if a Hopi family therapist were to treat the child of an Aristotelian parent. For the Hopi a language filled with predicates and few objects represents an outlook based on expectation and preparation for evolution and change. For the Aristotelian a language filled with nouns focuses on the things and the names of things as they are. Dell (1980b) develops these subtle epistemological differences in relation to questions of etiology and context when assessing the family theories of schizophrenia. He describes the Aristotelian/Newtonian paradigm, which characterizes traditional psychological models, as "a deterministic, cause-and-effect world in which the outcome of any set of events can be analyzed and predicted if only one knows beforehand the quantified characteristics of the objects involved" (p. 329). The alternative paradigm, "the epistemology of pattern . . . is oriented to shapes, forms, and relations [looking] not at objects themselves but at the 'pattern that connects' them'' (p. 329).

Something more fundamental than the words and the concepts they represent underlies the way that problems are defined and the differences that will be experienced in this process by the nosologist and by the family systems therapist.

WHAT IS THE BORDERLINE SYNDROME IN CHILDREN?

Current formulations of the genesis of borderline characteristics depend largely on object relations theory and the nature of the infant's internalization of objects to build a secure and reliable sense of self and non-self. Largely this process depends on the quality of the infant-mother interaction, "good enough" mothering, and the mother's capacity to provide an adequate holding environment (Winnicott, 1965) within which the infant can sort out the world of affectional objects.

Like many adult syndromes whose origins are supposed to be in childhood experience, the borderline syndrome takes on a different and rather confusing shape in childhood. Though the descriptive characteristics of impulsivity, affective storms, and fluctuating relationships with reality may be described in both the childhood syndrome and the adult syndromes, clinicians differ about the qualities of the borderline child, the origins, and the outcome of the syndrome in adulthood (Kestenbaum, 1983). Vela, Gottlieb and Gottlieb (1983, pp. 40-41) sought consensus on what was being described in the literature, and listed 6 characteristics of borderline children based on their reviews of all reports of borderline syndromes in children. These characteristics are summarized in Table I.

Pine (1983, pp. 90-97), on the other hand, emphasizes the more dynamic aspects of the syndrome in children, including those in Table II.

Yet a third way of understanding the borderline child is offered by Chethik (1986) who discusses the characteristic defects as summarized in Table III.

TABLE I. Consensus Symptoms for Borderline Conditions in Children

1. disturbed interpersonal relationships, characterized by:
   a. controlling, demanding,
   b. indiscriminate sociability or
   c. being extremely withdrawn and aloof,
   d. extreme outbursts of love or hate,
   e. exaggerated copying of another's behavior,
   f. isolation from peers and lack of friends.

2. disturbances in the sense of reality, characterized by:
   a. fantasies of being all-powerful, and behaving as if they were true
   b. extreme withdrawal into idiosyncratic fantasy
   c. difficulty differentiating play from reality
   d. paranoid ideation
   e. excessive use of magical thinking

3. excessive, intense anxiety, manifested by:
   a. chronic, constant, anxiety interfering with child's's functioning
   b. panic states
   c. anxiety about a wide variety of stimuli or new situations
   d. intense fear of separations

4. excessive and severe impulsive behavior resulting form minimal
   provocation, characterized by:
   a. repetitive fits of rage
   b. loss of control, e.g. destroying objects
   c. unmanagability due to aggressive behavior
   d. loss of contact with reality during these occasions
   e. tantrums lasting for an hour or more
   f. paranoid ideation during the tantrum

5. "neurotic-like" symptoms, e.g. rituals, somatic concerns, obsessions,
   multiple phobia, etc.

6. uneven or distorted development characterized by:
   a. deviant or erratic psysiologic patterning
   b. apathy, poor sucking, lack of responsiveness to human contact
   c. excessive rubbing, rolling, or head banging
   d. delay in motor or language areas

(From Vela, R.M., Gottlieb, E.H., and Gottlieb, H.P., Borderline Syndromes in Childhood: A critical review, in Robson, K.S., ed., The Borderline Child, New York: McGraw Hill, 1983, p. 40-41)

Borders and Boundaries

When thinking about ego weakness in the borderline syndrome, one necessarily thinks about the ego as a structure with borders which within the psyche differentiates it from the id and superego, and outside, differentiate self from other. Certain kinds of psychotic and borderline phenomena have been explained through using

TABLE II. Pine's Nosology of Borderline Syndrome in Children

1. shifting levels of ego organization, e.g. at one time being sensitively in touch with thoughts and feelings, in the next moment being out of contact with change in voice tome, affective expression, , etc.

2. internal disorganization in response to external disorganizers, relates to the children's attempts to handle and extremely chaotic environment internally

3. chronic ego deviance, e.g., panic, anxiety, unreliability of object attachment, self-object discrimination problems

4. incomplete internalization of psychosis

5. ego limitation,may remain in an early adaptive mode which interferes with later developments

(From Pine, F., A working nosology of borderline syndromes in childhood, in K.S. Robson, Ed., The Borderline Child, New York: McGraw Hill, 1983, 90-96)

TABLE III. Chethik's Description of Borderline Conditions in Childhood

1. instinctual defects, characterized by heightened aggressive drive, problems in the separation-individuation subphase, and problems in pregenital aggression related to physical illness in the first year of life.

2. ego defects, chracterized by problems in defense formation, prominant use of splitting, and primitive defenses of projection, devaluation, idealization, and denial

3. object relations defects, characterized by relating to objects on a need-gratifying basis, difficulty reaching the level of consistent object constancy, withdrawal into fantasy life with omnipotent, protective, need-satisfying objects, erection of self-objects, and interference with the process of constructive identification

4. developmental defects, characterized by a partial transition out of the stage of narcissism and many of the object relations defects described above

(From Chethik, M., (1986), Levels of borderline functioning in children: etiological and treatment considerations. Amer. J. Orthophyschiat. 56(1):109-110)

models of weak ego boundaries. Such notions of borders and boundaries lead to concrete pictures of fences, hedges, walls, and doors which delineate spaces and demarcate functions.

Boundary is also a family systems concept. Particularly in the Structural approach, boundary is an important abstraction referring to the negotiation of space and distance between individuals, subsystems, and systems. Furthermore, boundaries differentiate roles and functions within family systems. Thus boundaries, as family systems concepts, refer both to proximity and to hierarchy.

In researching family boundaries, Wood (1985) has defined aspects of family proximity and hierarchy, as on Table IV.

A wholistic expression of excessive proximity is in the concept of enmeshment, a notion of a high degree of family closeness, resonance between individuals and subsystems and unclear hierarchical functions, as well.

In Wood's schema "hierarchy" is the other function of family boundaries: the function of differentiating roles, tasks, and status within the family. Besides excessive proximity, another connotation of family enmeshment is role diffusion, poor hierarchical function, and cross-generational coalitions.

A rough translation of the concept of family boundaries into the language of ego psychology might go as follows: family boundaries are the way in which individual selves' interactions in the object world are regulated both from within and without. What this suggests, which differs from the usual theories about object relations theory and development of differentiation of self and other, is that the interaction between self and object world is constantly being regulated in the family; that it is not just a property of the individual's ego structure, formed in early life, and operational in later life, but it is a continuing process. Thus the translation of bounda-

TABLE IV. Family Boundaries

Proximity
CONTACT TIME
EMOTIONAL SPACE
PERSONAL SPACE
CONVERSATION SPACE
DECISION SPACE

Heirarchy
NURTURANCE
CONTROL
ALLIANCES
COALITIONS
PEERS

(From Wood, B., Proximity and hierarchy: orthogonal dimensions of family interconnectedness, Family Process, 24:487-507, 1986)

ries as concepts, from the realm of psychic structure to that of family systems leads to very different conclusions, because of the underlying differences in syntax, or epistemology.

FAMILY SYSTEMS AND FAMILY SYSTEMS

Family therapists differ in the degree to which they differentiate problems as being marital and family problems or as being primarily within individuals in which the family maintains or causes further dysfunction. But the family *systems* therapist finds that individual dysfunction is inseparable from its context, the family context being the most immediate. From the family systems perspective there can be no such thing as the borderline syndrome in an individual. It is not just a matter of having a different name or a different system of classifications. Different data are collected about a series of complaints, so that an entirely different set of conclusions will be drawn.

There are differences in approaches to family therapy. Some schools of family therapy are directly derived from psychodynamic theories. Practitioners of these approaches tend to use the family to correct or to mediate difficulties appreciated in the individual family member. These clinicians will identify and label the individual characteristics of all relevant individuals in the client system. The identified patient's symptoms may well be seen as the consequence of diagnosable psychopathology in significant family members. For example, a child with a borderline syndrome may have a mother with severe depression, or with borderline pathology, herself. Because of the identification of psychopathology and labelling of family members, the potential resources of the family tend to be negatively evaluated.

The family systems therapist sees the reality of human behavior as occurring in a relationship context. The family is the most immediate ecology of the child and is, therefore, the most accessible resource to the child. Tools of assessment for the family systems therapist include understanding of patterns and regulation of the context using general systems theory and cybernetics. Treatment involves mobilizing family systems resources in behalf of all of the family members.

CLASSICAL CASES:
TRADITIONAL AND FAMILY THERAPY

Since the borderline syndrome in childhood is a construct of psychodynamic theory, there is no adequate translation of the syndrome into family systems terms. A child who may meet the criteria for borderline syndrome in individual terms would not look the same in family terms. To illustrate this two classic cases from the literature which are presented as borderline will be discussed. Each will be presented briefly as they have been described; what family material is available will be presented, followed by hypotheses about the family system, an assessment, and a hypothetical family treatment plan.

"Velia" (Kestenbaum, 1983)

Velia presented at age 7 with poor academic achievement and poor social relationships with both teachers and peers. Problem behaviors included lying, stealing, fighting, and truancy.

Velia was born when her mother was 16 and her father was 17. The parents separated, and Velia lived till age 5 with her maternal grandparents. Velia's mother had left home when she was 15; her own father was an alcoholic, and her mother was a martyr member of a group who helped wives of alcoholics. Velia's mother remarried when she was 5, and Velia went to live with her mother and stepfather (see Figure 1). Adjustment difficulties were manifested in rages and sleepwalking. She also had severe difficulties getting along with other children.

Velia had two years of intensive individual therapy during which she manifested ambivalence towards the therapist.

My hypotheses about the family were that Velia was very attached to the grandparents, and they were very attached to her. It is even possible that her presence in the home brought the grandfather home, and he may have stopped drinking (this actually happened in a similar case). The grandparents experienced a great sense of loss when Velia went to live with her mother.

Furthermore, I believe that Velia's mother was very inexperienced and unsure of herself, and this insecurity was heightened by the fact that Velia was a vulnerable child. She was premature and clumsy, and she wore leg braces till 18 months of age. She also had

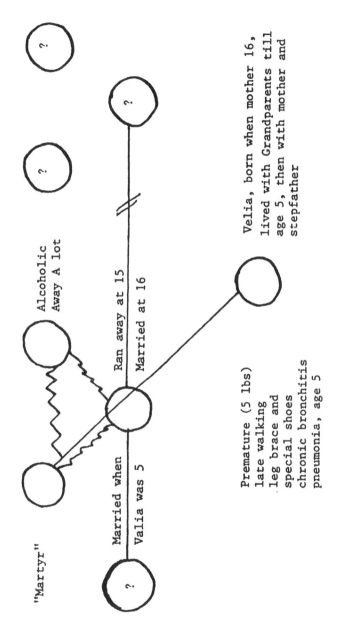

FIGURE 1. Velia Genogram

39

bronchitis as a young child. Velia's mother was further intimidated by the child's strong attachment to her grandparents and theirs to her.

Velia's stepfather must have been unclear about his role in relation to both the child and her mother.

Looked at this way, Velia's behavior maintained the system by reinforcing the mother's uncertainty and the stepfather's confusion, and thus sustaining the loyalty between herself and grandparents.

Based on these hypotheses, family treatment would include both mother and stepfather in sessions to see how they manage Velia and how they play with her. With the two parents present, the therapist would support management of Velia's behavior by getting them to make decisions about what is acceptable and insisting that they implement these decisions by containing her behavior in the sessions. Further, the therapist would create an opportunity for enjoyable play between parents and child in sessions.

It would be important to include the grandparents in some sessions to encourage ongoing relationships between them and the child and to clarify the different functions of parents and grandparents.

As Velia's behavior improved in the sessions, the therapist would help parents deal with Velia's school by giving them the necessary information to make decisions about her education and supporting collaboration between school personnel and parents to maintain consistency and clarity for Velia.

It is likely that there would be difficult struggles between parents and Velia which could result either in the mother's determination to care for her child with the mother prevailing by offering the child firm and clear limits, or in a decision to return Velia to the care of her grandparents, where the mother would continue to have an active role in decisions about health, education and welfare, a kind of joint custody arrangement.

"Matthew" (Chethik, 1986)

Matthew was 10 when he was hospitalized for withdrawal and impulsive, unprovoked outbursts.

About Matthew's early history it is reported that he cried constantly during his first year, often screaming without any known source of discomfort. The only way to soothe him was to drive endlessly in the family car. He was tense and stiff when held in his mother's arms. Later he was described as having severe tantrums and being quite uncontrollable, refusing to do anything for himself and requiring that his mother do everything for him.

No family history was given, but descriptions of the history and of Matthew's treatment indicated that he originally had two parents, and perhaps did at the time of treatment, as well. The mother was a central history giver and, as played out in his fantasy, was a central figure in Matthew's life, as was his little sister. A genogram represents how this comes across, as presented, with Matthew isolated in his context, and the father isolated in his (see Figure 2).

Little is described about Matthew's physical context prior to the hospitalization. Apparently this is regarded as irrelevant to the task of assessing and treating the child.

Matthew received daily psychoanalytic treatment for over two years in a hospital or residence with increasing home visits towards the latter part of his stay. He was finally discharged to public school. He continued to manifest extreme anxiety, unusual fears, and developed a set of what appears to be obsessive rituals to protect himself.

Some systems hypotheses would be that Matthew was a first

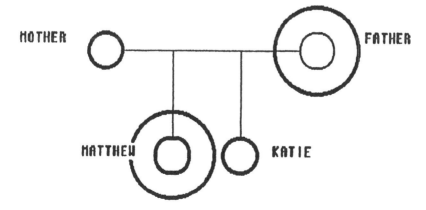

FIGURE 2. Matthew Family

child who was temperamentally extremely difficult. The parents who were quite young, had many conflicts about how to calm the child down which resulted in a kind of estrangement where the father spent more and more time away from the home, leaving the mother to cope with Matthew, by herself. Matthew's difficulties increased with the birth of his sister, Katie, who was easier for both parents to handle. Matthew's mother continued to be extremely involved with him to protect him from his father's extreme disappointment and irritation.

Matthew first entered treatment when he was 5, with a child psychiatrist who saw him frequently. A social worker saw his mother; no one spoke with the father. Matthew was admitted to a therapeutic school. Generally the mother felt responsible for Matthew, and she was intensely relieved when hospitalization was suggested when he was 10.

Katie developed without incident, a real joy to both her parents.

Based on these hypotheses, family treatment could have begun with the pediatrician, observing that these parents have an extremely difficult child. The pediatrician would offer three things: support and the information that the child is difficult, and it is not the parents' fault; involvement of the father in a plan which spells the mother and helps him to feel useful and competent with his child; and sedative medication in judicial amounts for the infant to give the parents some relief.

If difficulties persisted, the family would be referred to a family oriented child psychiatrist who would continue the above plan and add an element of psychoeducation, focusing the parents on the child's development, his increasing grasp of his world, and his increasing competence. The parents would be closely involved with each other and their child. They would appreciate themselves as parents who have dealt with a more difficult than average infant, and they would be proud of the talented and capable youngster they would see growing up with them.

If family therapy were initiated later, at age 10, for example, it might go like this. The entire family including both children and both parents would be seen. After a session of observation and data collection, the therapist would observe that Matthew was provocatively and determinedly isolating himself from the other family members, who seemed to be helpless about this. An activity would be selected which capitalized on Matthew's skills (cartoons) and the family would be set to work to create a joint cartoon which tells a story about the family. During this project the family would be helped to collaborate, to acknowledge each other's place in the family and each other's skills. The parents would be encouraged to manage the project, to deal with Matthew's attempts to withdraw from the group and with Katie's provocation of Matthew. This project could take several months.

Other family activities would be planned (by the family) within the therapy sessions in such a way that everyone would be included in the planning.

Matthew's adjustment in school would be considered, and parents would be supported in their inquiries about the appropriateness of the academic and social environment for their son.

In the end, the parents could become sufficiently confident of their own expertise for their gifted, but eccentric son that they could advocate for him in education and help him to negotiate what is likely to be a very difficult social life.

THE FAMILY THERAPY PORTFOLIO

The next two cases are from the practices of family therapists. They have been selected because they presented with very disturbing symptoms which descriptively fit the criteria for the borderline syndrome in childhood, although this is not how they were assessed by the therapists; nor is it how they were treated.

"Vincenzo"

Vincenzo, called Greg, first presented to me at age 4 1/2 in the midst of a visitation conflict between his parents. Greg's disturbing behaviors included outbursts of anger, including tantrums, destroying things, throwing things at people whom he also loved, sleep disturbance, aggressive behavior, foul language, and some sexual preoccupations including excessive masturbation, attempts to put his penis into the mouth of a Yorkshire terrier, and attempts at anal intercourse with a neighbor's 5-year-old child.

Greg was the only child of his young parents who had never married. His mother had been physically abused by his father, had finally left, gone into hiding with Greg, and had finally gone to live with her mother and stepfather. For several months the mother had brought the child for Sunday afternoon visits with the father, but this arrangement deteriorated when the mother went to court for child-support and the father responded by suing for overnight visitation. Both parties won, and the child began to have overnight visits with the father which often included his new girlfriend. It is not at all clear what went on during these visits; the child reports sleeping in bed with his father and girlfriend and watching pornographic movies. His own room was being used to raise puppies, and he referred to it as "the shit room." It was at this time that he exploded into his use of foul language and sexual anxieties, so his mother finally discontinued the visits. A series of "accidents" were attrib-uted to the father, and the court battle raged on.

The father, Vincenzo, called Vinnie, came from an ethnically Italian family and was a physically attractive, muscular man involved in body building and currently employed in running his own gym. His own father was involved in "business" of various types. There were gas stations and other "fronts," but drug dealing was suspected, and he was a known philanderer. In fact, it is said that he had two wives who lived in houses on parallel streets separated by a back fence. Vinnie insisted on calling his son "Vinnie." He had one older sister who was strung out on cocaine, a loyal but tense attachment to his father, and, to his mother, he could do no wrong. He was very clear about his machismo and anxious to convey the same attitudes to his son. Thus he told him not to talk to "foggy" psychiatrists, to use macho four-letter words, and to be disdainful of sissy institutions, like schools.

Greg's mother, Kathy, was the second of three children whose parents split up when she was 7. Her family was ethnically Irish. Her father was an alcoholic, and she often used to find him in bars and take him home, especially after her parents split up. Her mother struggled to make enough money for the three kids and was often exhausted and irritable with them. The oldest boy was the peace-maker with his mother, Kathy tried to protect her father, and the youngest was the baby. When Kathy was 12, her mother, Marie, began to work as a secretary for a successful small business man who was deformed with severe kyphosis. She began dating him when Kathy was 14, and married him when she was 24. He, too, was Italian, his name is Gregory. The child was named "Vincenzo Gregory." Kathy was a good student but distractible and "hungry," thus very vulnerable to the attractions of Vinnie with his high life-style and lavish affection. For a year prior to seeing me Kathy had been in psychotherapy for eating disorders and depression. At the time she came to me, both were under control without medication. See Figure 3 for Greg's genogram.

Greg lived with his mother and her mother and stepfather (Marie and Gregory). His aunt Leanne also lived there. The grandparents offered a great deal of financial support for Kathy and emotional support in her struggle with Vinnie, but they had the expectation that she would manage Greg, even though they believed that he was emotionally disturbed and need psychiatric help. The mother was expected to manage Greg, and the other family members had a hands-off policy about his discipline, though they lavished toys and special things upon him.

Greg was not allowed to visit with his father, at all, until the court case was settled. He very much missed him and felt that he was responsible for not being able to see his father. He was torn in his attachment to his mother and the disloyalty to his father that this implied. Thus, though his mother called him "Greg," he thought he would prefer to be called "Vinnie" because that was his father's name.

It was recommended to the Court that Greg see his father under supervised and managed circumstances, to foster the relationship between father and son but to minimize the clash in values and expectations between the father's family and mother's family. The father was instructed to call his son "Greg," and to visit with him in a therapeutic preschool which involved parents in the curriculum. Thus Vinnie could see his son on a weekly basis. At the same time treatment was ongoing with Greg and Kathy, with Marie and Gregory attending sessions periodically (efforts to involve Vinnie in the treatment were thwarted for a variety of reasons).

One hypothesis was that Greg was involved in a loyalty struggle which was heightened by the different values systems of each side.

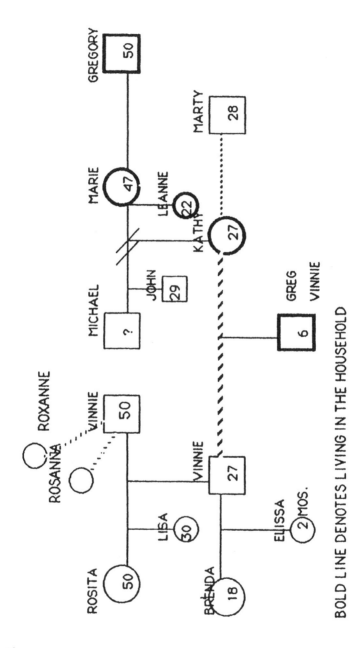

FIGURE 3. Vincenzo Family

BOLD LINE DENOTES LIVING IN THE HOUSEHOLD

His mother and her family valued (perhaps revered) education and professional status, and attempted to each Greg to be respectful, loving, and polite. His father and his family valued independence and personal success and devalued education and societal institutions. The names, Vinnie and Greg, reflected these two different realities.

A second hypothesis was that in his mother's home everyone saw him as emotionally disturbed, and they tended to excuse his behavior on that basis. While they wished for him to behave in a certain fashion, no one felt that they could expect him to do so.

A third hypothesis was that there were further differences in management and expectations between the grandparents and aunt and the mother.

Treatment began with the maternal household to clarify what was wrong with Greg—not an illness, but confusion and lack of clear, firm, control. This was demonstrated by my own strong, affectionate management of his aggressive behavior in the office, to which he responded by loud protest and kicking, but ultimately yielded affectionately to my successful restraint of him. At first his mother and grandparents looked on in fear for me. Later his mother undertook the same management.

In sessions Greg and his mother would play together, working on collaboration and appreciating his competence in activities which ranged from drawing, wrestling, admiring various feats of his prowess (e.g., jumping from one chair to another across greater and greater spans), and building block towers to be knocked down by various characters from the Superfriends and the Masters of the Universe. During these sessions the mother was in charge of keeping Greg's behavior within acceptable limits.

Parts of the office were off-limits because of my "personal stuff" and many behaviors were off-limits as well.

Greg's grandparents returned for another round when Greg's behavior at home exploded. The differences between the adults managing Greg were discussed, and consistency from all the adults in the family was advocated, and they developed an agreed upon response to unacceptable behaviors (such as breaking toys, using foul language, hitting people, and torturing the dogs), a response which would be implemented by any adult who witnessed the behaviors. There was a striking improvement after this.

The treatment of Greg's family was complicated by their reverence for professionals, and they had many in their lives. Thus without active coordination of the teachers and other doctors in his life other explanations for his behavior were sought and accepted and some of the consistency and firmness with him slipped, as did his behavior. Furthermore, the massive differences between father and mother persisted. After he graduated from the therapeutic preschool, Greg did not see his father, at all, because Vinnie did not take steps to develop another plan for visitation which was acceptable to the Court. In the meantime Vinnie married his girlfriend, and they had a baby. The task for Greg's mother in the context of these changes with people with whom Greg wasn't in contact was to maintain consistency, love, and appreciation for Greg in an atmosphere of sympathy and understanding of his feeling for his father.

"Rachel"

Rachel was 10 when she presented to me for family therapy. She had previously been in individual therapy for two years for a school phobia, which had improved to the extent that her therapist had recommended that she go to overnight camp. Her parents arranged for this in spite of the fact that they did not feel that it was a good thing to do. Rachel was miserable from the start and begged to come home. Her parents consulted the therapist who told them to make a deal that if she participated in camp activities until parents' visiting day, they would bring her home. They did, and Rachel began to manifest symptoms of severe obsessive and phobic nature. She constantly demanded reassurance that she was not going to die, performed all sorts of rituals around eating, bathing, and, eventually, ambulating, which progressively paralyzed her so that her mother was having to feed, dress, and bathe her. She also developed such fears about food that she would spit it out and even attempt to clean her saliva. She was unable to sleep and kept her mother up all night to be sure that she didn't fall asleep and die.

Rachel was the younger of two girls whose parents were separated when she was a small infant and divorced soon afterwards.

Though moved to another state, the father kept in contact with his children, but, as Rachel grew older, her father's contacts with her made her so anxious that he eventually stopped seeing her and simply spoke with her on the phone weekly. Rachel's mother had been raised in a wealthy, indulgent family which did value education; she had a bachelor's degree in social work and worked as a counsellor. Both of the maternal grandparents were dead, and the mother's only brother was in a distant state. The father was remarried, but Rachel had no relationship with her stepmother. Two years prior to our contacts Rachel's mother, Jan, married David, a divorced father of one, an attorney. It was at this time that Rachel's clinginess escalated into full-blown separation anxiety symptoms, and her therapy had begun. At that time Rachel was evaluated by the school psychologist who found her functioning in the bright average range of 10. She noted marked "performance anxiety." At the time of David's marriage to Jan, his mother was dying in a nursing home. She actually died in the spring of the year that Rachel made her fateful trip to camp. Figure 4 shows Rachel's genogram.

Rachel lived with her mother and stepfather. Her mother had just finished her master's degree in social work, having worked on it for five years. Her older sister, Annelise, was a student at a nearby university. Rachel was an average student academically, was reasonably comfortable in school, but had no friends after school. She regarded herself as the class clown.

Rachel's parents had been in marital therapy with a psychiatrist who had also been giving antidepressants to David. David reported that he had been suicidal; stating that several months ago he had sat with a gun in his lap, trying to decide whether or not to shoot himself.

For the previous two years Rachel had been in individual therapy with a psychologist. Her parents consulted the psychologist who directed them about how to handle Rachel's fears and symptoms. The parents had depended upon the psychologist to direct them about what to do with Rachel.

Our first hypothesis was that Rachel was very attached to her mother and vice versa; for at a time when Rachel's mother was separated and on her own, for the first time in her life, Rachel was someone who gave meaning to her. As Rachel grew older, both she

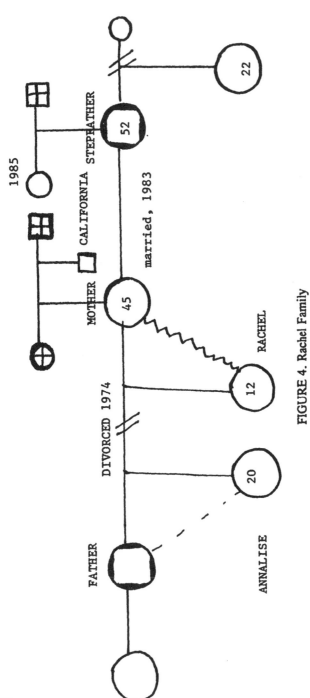

FIGURE 4. Rachel Family

and her mother became increasingly and ambivalently independent of one another—Rachel to school, mother, also to school, and into a new marriage. This separation was not without difficulty, manifested mostly by Rachel's symptoms, but also by David's isolation and despair.

Our second hypothesis was that as Rachel became more involved with her therapist, and the therapist became more authoritative, the parents lost more of their confidence about making decisions on her behalf.

In the first family session Rachel insisted on having the session focused on her, becoming very angry when the therapist talked about anything else. Finally she threatened to pull the family out of therapy, saying, "This isn't helping me."

She did not do her ritual behavior in the session, but she was extremely anxious, unable to sit still and barely able to sit, at all. The therapist concentrated on getting to know the family, inquiring about their attempts to cope with the problems, and their theories about them. Rachel's mother at first thought of her daughter as ill but then admitted that the child's behavior was irritating and frustrating, as well as disgusting. David put forth a theory that Rachel's death fears may have come from her death wishes against her mother; then noted the overcloseness between the two.

The parents were encouraged to manage Rachel's difficulties. During the session Rachel was asked to wait in the waiting room while the parents consulted with the therapist. The therapist wanted to empower the parents with magic over the magic experienced by Rachel. Together they hit upon the idea of giving Rachel a magic phrase that was to have occurred to Jan in a dream. The dream was that God told Jan to ask David for a magic phrase. David supplied the phrase, inter alia, and Jan and he told Rachel to say the phrase every time she experienced the compulsion to do one of her rituals or ask for reassurance about death. They also decided what they would expect from Rachel in terms of eating, dressing, etc.

Work in the ongoing family sessions was on clarifying the family system and relationships. A discussion of finances and management of money, for example, focused clearly on their circumstances and how the family actually functioned, in a somewhat haphazard fashion.

Questions were raised about where did Rachel, rather than David, fit in to the family. Relationships between Rachel and her sister and her father were also explored. All of these areas clarify family boundaries in terms of roles, hierarchy, and proximity.

Rachel demonstrated immediate improvement from the most distressing symptoms, and after 12 sessions she was doing quite well. She has no rituals and no obvious fears, except on Tuesdays prior to her therapy sessions. In the car on the way to the session, she would bring up things like a cut finger, and ask her parents whether they thought she will survive. She was also doing well in school, had had friends over for a pajama party, and had been to sleep overs at friends' houses. There were still many areas of family boundaries to straighten out in the family, both between Jan and David and between their family and their former spouses. Rachel kept a watchful eye on them, and the therapists were aware that if Jan and David slipped up, Rachel was ready to rescue.

SUMMARY

All of these examples, hypothetical (from the literature) or real, illustrate that these children, who might be characterized as having the borderline syndrome are difficult individuals who live in very complicated families. These children were constitutionally intense and demanding individuals and lived in systems in which there was confusion about roles and function. This was particularly true of parenting functions in the families of Velia, Greg, and Rachel. In Matthew's case, the relationship between the hospital/therapeutic staff and the parenting functions was undoubtedly confusing to both him and his parents. Recognizing the extraordinary efforts required to manage a difficult child, the family therapist must help the parent figures organize themselves to provide consistency and limits, as well as recognition and appreciation of the child's assets. Thus a focus on the child's skills and playfulness can be a useful context for introducing structure into the family system.

Work with these families may go on longer than much family work with child problems because of the system's tendency to become disorganized, often in response to a challenge by the child or by another system in which the child has become involved (such as the school or another professional system). A long-term relationship with the therapist can be helpful even though the family may not have to attend regular sessions over this time. It is essential, however, that the therapist maintain consistent expectations both of the child and the parents.

CONCLUSION

The concept of the borderline syndrome in childhood has been largely based on a concept of ego functioning and maintenance of ego boundaries. Thus it is a psychodynamically conceptualized syndrome. Family systems theory focuses on interpersonal space, and thus can adopt the concept of boundaries as they are manifested in proximity, role differentiation, and maintenance of hierarchy. As we have seen, children who have been described as borderline appear to live in families where there is considerable confusion about these aspects of boundaries. Treatment aimed at clarifying parent child hierarchy, clarifying intra- and extrafamilial boundaries, and clarifying roles within the family can result in rapid abatement of the worst symptoms and maintain the family intact while supporting the increasing competence of natural family resources.

REFERENCES

Chethik, M. (1986), Levels of borderline functioning in children: etiological and treatment considerations. *Amer. J. Orthopsychiat.*, 56(1):109-119.

Dell, P.F. (1980a), The Hopi family therapist and the Aristotelian parents. *J. Marital and Family Therapy*, 123-130.

Dell, P.F. (1980b), Researching the family theories of schizophrenia: an exercise in epistemological confusion. *Family Process*, 19(4):321-335.

Kestenbaum, C.J. (1983), The borderline child at risk for major psychiatric disorder in adult life, in K.S. Robson, ed., *The Borderline Child: Approaches to Etiology, Diagnosis, and Treatment*. New York: McGraw Hill, 49-82.

Pine, F. (1983), A working nosology of borderline syndromes in childhood, in K.S. Robson, ed., *op. cit.*, 83-100.

Shapiro, T. (1983), The borderline syndrome in children: a critique, in K.S. Robson, ed., *op. cit.*, 11-29.

Vela, R., Gottlieb, H., Gottlieb, E. (1983), Borderline syndromes in childhood: a critical review, in K.S. Robson, ed., *op. cit.*, 31-48.

Winnicott, D.W. (1965), *The Maturational Process and the Facilitating Environment: Studies in the Theory of Emotional Development*. New York: International Universities Press.

Wood, B. (1985), Proximity and hierarchy: orthogonal dimensions of family interconnectedness. *Family Process*, 24:487-507.

Systemic Family Therapy with Young Children and Their Families: Use of the Reflecting Team

William D. Lax

This paper addresses two issues: the inclusion of young children in family therapy and a discussion of a systemic approach called the "reflecting team" (Andersen, 1987). After a theoretical presentation, case examples will be utilized to discuss how the reflecting team incorporates young children's participation in clinical interviews as integral components of the therapy system.

INTRODUCTION

Family therapists and theorists have recognized and discussed all stages of the family life-cycle including the time in the family life-cycle when there are young children in the family and the transitions that take place for all family members (Carter & McGoldrick, 1980; Haley, 1973; Zilbach, 1974, 1987; Zilbach, Bergel & Gass, 1968, 1972). Unfortunately, young children who are part of the family system coming to therapy are often left out of the treatment. Children are sometimes dismissed as not being full members of a family (Dowling & Jones, 1978), may be viewed as "distracting" and will "impede the work" which needs to be done (Verheij,

William D. Lax, MD, is Director of the Brattleboro Family Institute.

The author expresses deep appreciation to Lynn Hoffman, ACSW, and Tom Andersen, MD, for their invaluable roles in the development of my thinking and the formulation of the ideas included in this paper. Also thanks to her colleagues Judy Davidson, MA, Dario J. Lussardi, MA, Dusty Miller, EdD, and Margaret Ratheau, MA, at the Brattleboro Family Institute who have helped expand her thinking and applications of this model.

1980), or therapists may have difficulties keeping young children involved in ongoing therapy (Wolfe & Collins, 1983).

Recently several authors have begun to discuss the importance of including young children in the therapy process. In addition they have suggested theoretical perspectives and methods which would facilitate this process (Bloch, 1976; Combrinck-Graham, 1986; Maloney, 1981; Zilbach, 1986).

One newer model that includes young children in the therapy process is the "reflecting team" (Andersen, 1987). It is an expansion of the systemic model originally developed by the Milan Associates and is an expression of the "new epistemology" in family therapy (see Boscolo, Cecchin, Hoffman & Penn, 1987; MacKinnon & Miller, 1987). This model maintains some basic assumptions which have evolved from the work of several family therapy theorists and other authors in related fields (Anderson, Goolishian & Winderman, 1986; Bogdan, 1984; von Foerster, 1981; von Glasersfeld, 1984; Hoffman, 1986, 1987). Some of these theoretical guidelines are as follows:

1. Problems are viewed as existing in the domain of meanings and are an "ecology of ideas";
2. Problems generate systems rather than systems create problems and cases are seen as "problem determined systems";
3. People cannot leave the field or change under a negative connotation: emphasis is on positive or logical connotation;
4. There is a recursive relationship between meanings and action: as meanings change, behaviors may be altered;
5. Reality is observer defined, and the model ascribes to a "second order cybernetics" in which the therapist is a participant in the construction of the therapy system's "reality";
6. Since the therapist can only make his/her own constructions of the problem system (of which the therapist is a part) there are no right views, but only ones that "fit" the system and are acceptable to it;
7. There is an emphasis on sharing of information versus withholding;
8. Therapy is viewed as maintaining a lateral position between therapist and client rather than a hierarchical one.

Further Theoretical Considerations

Andersen and his colleagues' development of the "reflecting team" model has been strongly influenced by the work and writings of Bateson, Boscolo, Cecchin, Goolishian, Hoffman, Maturana, and Penn. As will be described later in this paper, the reflecting team format is a recursive one with conversations folding back upon one another, like the kneading of bread dough, continually incorporating new distinctions. This attention to recursive processes has been influenced by the field of cybernetics.

Cybernetics developed from the work of Norbert Weiner (1961) and includes concepts such as homeostasis, self-regulation and self-organization. It was viewed as a science of "observed systems." As the field developed, it underwent a "second order" shift, with the addition of von Foerster's ideas of a "cybernetics of cybernetics." These included concepts of autonomy, self-reference and responsibility. Von Foerster described this shift in the field of cybernetics as a movement to the science of "observing systems."

This second order cybernetics was further influenced by a strain of thinking called radical constructivism. These ideas propose that our knowledge of the world is based on our own ordering and organizing of our perceptions and is not based upon or validated by an external reality (von Glasersfeld, 1984; Steier & Smith, 1985). As describers of this world, we are part of an "observing system." We make these observations within a context in which our observations make "sense" to us. All distinctions are "valid" with reality determined through an agreement among a community of observers. Thus, the world is a "multiverse" of views with all views being constructed (Maturana, 1984).

Anderson, Goolishian and Winderman (1986) have expanded these ideas and applied them directly to the field of family therapy. They suggested that problems occur in language and may "exist simply because someone says 'this is a problem,' and has the authority to enforce response and action" (Anderson, Goolishian & Winderman, 1986, p. 7). People and patterns may develop around these problems to form a "system" which is held together through their common language, distinctions, and social constructs.

Problem resolution or change of this pattern is facilitated by the therapist attending to the recursive organization of this "system of meanings" and assisting the system to generate new meanings. It is this shift in view which will alter the problem and/or facilitate change. The process of the reflecting team is one approach that assists this shift in meaning.

THE REFLECTING TEAM

People can only participate in a conversation to the extent of their own repertoire of interactions and ideas. These ideas are constructed and known through our drawing distinctions or perceiving differences in the world (Andersen, 1987; Bateson, 1972; Maturana, 1984).

A stuck family system is thus limited by its range of ideas and meanings and needs new ideas in order to further evolve. These new ideas, distinctions or differences which facilitate change must fit with the family system. As Bateson described them, they must be a "difference that makes a difference" (1972, p. 453). Andersen expanded Bateson's understanding of differences, describing three different kinds of differences. The first kind are differences that are so small that they do not make any difference in the family system. These differences may be too similar to the family's view or repertoire and may not even by noticed. The second kind of differences are ones that are so different from the family's view that they will not make a difference. These differences are too foreign to the problem system to be acceptable. The third kind are differences that are just different enough from the family's current repertoire, being neither too similar nor too foreign, to make a difference leading to change.

Andersen changes the world difference to "usual" and "unusual." He believes that if people are interacting in too usual a pattern there may, at times, be little room for change or development. On the other hand, if they are relating to one another in a way that is too unusual for one another, the conversation stops. Our job as family therapists is to try to participate in conversations with families and generate the third kind of differences which will potentially make a difference in the problem system.

The Interview and Reflections

The therapeutic approach with a "reflecting team" is a process in which a team, either behind the one-way screen or in the room, watches and listens to the interviewer's conversation with the "stuck" family system. At some point in the interview, the therapist and family stop their interview: they then watch and listen to the reflecting team discuss their perceptions and explanations regarding the interview and the stuck system. When the team has completed their comments, the family and therapist resume their conversation and discuss the thoughts presented by the team, with the team again observing this conversation.[1]

Differences are introduced within the therapeutic interview/conversation through the use of questions and as "reflections" about the system, the therapist and/or the interview as a whole.

The interview between the therapist and the family follows the questioning model first introduced by the Milan Associates and which has been discussed by Penn (1982, 1985) and Tomm (1985). This approach uses direct and circular questions to elicit "information" about the family system. A focus of this process is to determine the distinctions or "pictures" that are drawn within the family system. Particular attention is made not to ask questions that are too radically different from the family system's usual mode of interacting. For example, with a family that believes "children are to be seen and not heard," it would be too unusual to initially ask the children about their parent's relationship.

The interviewer stays "close" to the family, attending to what is important to them and what they present in the interview. She attempts to maintain a neutral position to the participants and their views during the conversation, and to look for openings to follow and opportunities to introduce new distinctions. With the team behind the one-way mirror during the interview, the therapist is able to fully participate, uninterrupted, in the therapy conversation.

It is during the reflecting part of the session that the team can comment on the interview and introduce views of their own. There are two kinds of reflections that a team may present to the stuck family system: "mirroring" and "speculating" (M. Hald, personal communication, April 20, 1987). Mirroring includes reflecting back to the family what was observed both verbally and non-verbally, including taking a family member's seat, reporting on his or her activity during the meeting, and assuming postures, gestures, tone, pace and language of different family members. Speculating includes reflecting back hypotheses, "interpretations," metaphors, homework assignments, comments on the therapist's actions during the interview, and raising questions that were not introduced during the meeting. Reflections highlight possible underlying premises (Bateson, 1972), "reference values" (Powers, 1973), "cognitive schemata" (Neisser, 1976) or "Karmic issues" (L. Hoffman, personal communication, September 29, 1987) as well as specific behavioral interactions and patterns.

In addition, there are several rules of thumb that may serve as guidelines for the reflecting team. These include but are not restricted to the following:

1. Comments are formed as positive or logical connotations as opposed to negative attributions or blaming;
2. Speculations are restricted to the conversations that have taken place in the room. Prior information obtained from referral sources or other outside contacts are excluded from the reflecting team's comments;
3. Comments attend to both verbal and non-verbal communications. What is seen and heard is often highlighted through the mirror, so team members must be respectful with their comments;
4. Reflections should attempt to present both sides of the dilemma, moving from an either/or position to a both/and or neither/nor position;
5. Emphasis is on presenting a "smorgasbord of ideas" versus "correct" interpretations;
6. Ideas should be presented tentatively, with qualifiers such as "I was wondering," "perhaps," "possibly," or "it's just an idea";
7. Comments and questions may be raised which the therapist did not or could not say in the interview. This can include comments on "difficult" topics, such as alcohol/substance abuse,

suspected incest, and violence, which were not raised during the interview.

THE ROLE OF YOUNG CHILDREN IN THE THERAPY

Since this model works with the "meaningful system" (Imber-Coppersmith, 1985) or system of meanings, young children are seen as participants in the conversation regarding the problem. Whether the interaction or conversation is verbal or non-verbal, children can be useful participants. They contribute to the meetings in a variety of ways as Zilbach (1986) has noted in her discussion of "critical functions" in the roles of young children in family therapy. Children have a view of the situation which, while not necessarily expressed in a verbal way, may bring family issues to the surface or serve as an index of the group affect (Dowling, 1978). Their views, expressed in play, comments, drawings, metaphor, or pantomime can offer the therapist a different picture of the family dynamics or interchange within the consulting room. Sometimes their presence alone, coupled with the family's interactions with them, can greatly facilitate the therapy process. An example of this can be seen in the following case.

In the initial telephone call Mrs. Ryan stated that she and her husband wanted to resolve "some difficulties" between them. She said they had been in therapy before, both individually and as a couple, and found it very useful for this process. At the initial interview both agreed that it had been Mrs. Ryan's idea to seek out therapy at this time. She feared that the two of them would become absorbed with their four-month-old child who would then come between them. She believed that they would lose their connection to one another over time, and when their son would leave home they would separate. While Mr. Ryan agreed that there had been difficulties in the past, he could not understand his wife's concerns or how their son could possibly come between them and threaten their relationship.

The interview was filled with confusion regarding what they felt their difficulties were or would be in the future. They both alluded to "control" issues in the past regarding issues of health and personal independence. They explained how they would get into extended discussions with one another trying to convince the other of their position. These would turn into a cold war with each going their separate ways. Neither was able to understand the other's position, now or in the past. The interview seemed to follow the couple's former (and present) pattern of discussions: they became increasingly frustrated with one another and conversation became more difficult.

The Ryans came to the second interview with their son. They still did not understand what the other was talking about regarding current or past issues. Shortly into the session, their son began to cough. As the discussion between Mr. and Mrs. Ryan began to become more exasperating, their son continued to cough more and Mr. Ryan picked him up and placed him on his knee in front of him. He noticed that his wife changed her expression, and he explained that the coughing was a natural reaction on the child's part. Mrs. Ryan offered another explanation and began a lengthy discussion of diet, health, and the implications for their son's coughing. Their discussion about the child escalated until Mrs. Ryan stopped and said "See, this is exactly what happens. One of us is always placing him in between us. Don't you see what we're doing?" Both were silent for a moment and slowly began a discussion of *how* they had been arguing, without the focus on *what* they had been arguing about. They commented how they both felt they had used their son as a buffer between the two of them. Both reported that this moment reminded them of their own parents and of feelings each had growing up.

They let the therapist hold the child while they continued this conversation, which was filled with lengthy elaborations of their families of origin. Both described having overbearing parents and developing ways to shut them out of their lives. They had carried many ideas from their own families into this marriage, vowing never to be overridden again or to do that to their child. They considered how "not understanding" was also a way of protecting themselves from being overridden. The remainder of the therapy focused on underlying vows or premises regarding these issues and how they affected the marriage.

The inclusion of their young son greatly facilitated the treatment process. Through their interactions with the child in the room, each was able to make different distinctions both to themselves and to the other regarding behaviors around the child. They were able to become observers to their own process and have a different kind of conversation than they had before. The blaming connotation of "not understanding" was removed, with their behavior toward one another "making sense," given each's personal history. They were now able to view each other from a new perspective, feeling relieved that the other truly understood and could provide opportunities to "work through" old personal issues.

In many instances when young children express their views, verbally and non-verbally, these opinions may not be as reified or well formed as adults. Like their parents, they may be under constraints regarding what can be said due to the complexity of relationships within the family. However, young children still maintain a greater freedom of action than adults, and they can offer valuable distinctions to the therapeutic conversation. The therapist may then have a better "picture" of the family's view of their dilemma and will be able to construct his/her own descriptions of their system based on more information.

Regardless of reasons offered by parents, therapists or referring persons for exclusion of young children in treatment, they are unavoidably a part of the ongoing system which surrounds the presenting or underlying problem.

The following are case examples of the use of the reflecting team with families with young children.

The Hurling Son

Mrs. Hunter called, stating that her daughter was "defiant" and would not listen to her. The family included her husband (37) and herself (35), two daughters, Kim (14) and Debbie (8), and a son, Mike (6). All family members came to the initial appointment. Mr. Hunter made it clear that coming was his wife's idea, and he did not have any difficulties with his daughter. He said that they were close, and she was just as "sweet and thoughtful as she had always been." He could not understand his wife's difficulties with her. The younger daughter agreed with her mother, that Kim spites her mother any time she can and while she does not refuse to "sit" for her and her brother, Kim always puts up a lengthy vocal argument about having to do it.

Kim stated that her mother treated her like a "slave," always asking her to take care of the younger two kids. She resented her mother and felt that she was treated like an infant on some occasions, yet asked to be "grown-up" and assume responsibilities of the oldest child on others. She stated that she could not wait until she was 18 when she could leave home.

Mr. Hunter agreed that he treated her differently than his wife did, as he did not make as many demands of her as she did. At this point the parents were clearly in disagreement as to whether Kim was demonstrating difficulties or not.

This discussion between the parents became more intense, with both arguing whether there was a "problem" or not. When the conversation had reached a point where it appeared that Mr. Hunter's view would prevail over the family and the problems would be minimized, Mike, who had been quietly playing on the floor with some Legos, got up, ran across the room and hurled himself into the corner of a TV monitor that was on the floor. His head was cut and bleeding. Mrs. Hunter and Kim both ran over to him, picked him up and after examining his head took him to a bathroom out in the hall. Mr. Hunter did not move from his seat, look distressed or at any time attend to his son.

When Mike and his mother were ready to return to the room the reflecting team said that they had some comments that they would like to make. The family and therapist switched places with the team: the team came into the consulting room while the therapist and the family moved into the observation room so they could watch and listen to the team's comments. The reflecting team began with some comments about Mike's actions and raised questions about the family's explanation of his behavior: was this usual for him to act in this way or more typical of the other children. They complimented the family on being able to both stay cool and attend to the situation and wondered whether it was usual for Mrs. Hunter to care for all of them. Were there any disagreements about how she was raising the children up to this point, and were the parents in agreement regarding the children's future plans and well-being.

When the team finished their reflections they returned to the observation room, and the therapist and family came back into the consulting room. Mr. Hunter began talking immediately, saying that this was not typical of Mike, as he was more like himself, "reserved and predictable." He said that he and his wife had the same long-range plans for their children and both had their children's best interests at heart. There *were* problems that needed attention, one of which was that he and his wife had different views on some issues. He reported that until recently they had been in agreement on almost everything that concerned themselves and the children. Now they had some "small" differences. Both parents agreed that Mrs. Hunter was having troubles with Kim, that Kim's grades were starting to drop at school, and that she was not as "social" as she had been in the past. Both parents and the children agreed to return for a second appointment.

The next meeting began with a brief discussion of their "small" differences and how these developed. Mrs. Hunter described how she and her husband had very different backgrounds. She was the oldest child from a family of three children. Her father, a factory worker, died when she was very young, and she and her mother shared the responsibilities of the other two children. She was often left alone with her siblings while her mother was at work and learned to be very "responsible." Mr. Hunter was the youngest of two children. His parents were professionals, and he had very few responsibilities at home regarding his brother or the household.

The parents stated that they had conflicting expectations of Kim, due to these different backgrounds. Mr. Hunter said he often related to her as a younger child than she was and thought that it was fine for her to stay young and not grow up so fast. He liked playing with her and stated that "she keeps me feeling young." Mrs. Hunter, on the other hand, thought Kim should have even more responsibilities at home. Kim was confused!

Both parents agreed that Mrs. Hunter first started to notice difficulties at about the same time that she had considered going back to work. At that time all of the children were in school, and she had much more free time than she wished to have. Mr. Hunter did not like this idea, as he felt that she should be available to her children at all times, particularly when they came home from school. When

Mrs. Hunter started to have difficulty with Kim she had given up the idea of returning to work.

The family and therapist switched places with the reflecting team, with the team coming into the consulting room and the therapist and family going into the observation room. The team discussed several ideas. Since Kim and her father were so close, perhaps she may be "voicing" her father's thoughts and wishes about her mother's returning to work. He was not the kind of man who would openly disagree with or "forbid" his wife from doing what she wanted. Also, perhaps each parent was being loyal to their own families by raising their children as they had been raised.

One team member thought that it might be best to focus on the problem with which they were all concerned and presenting to us: Kim's problems. The team considered the dilemma from Kim's perspective as well as the parents': with each parent having a different view, much confusion must exist regarding how old Kim might feel and act at different times. She would hear "be older" from her mother and "be younger" from her father. Another team member suggested that the problem which the parents faced may mirror their ambivalence and desires regarding their own issues of growing up: father wanted to be able to act younger with Kim and mother wanted her to grow up and go to work!

After switching places with the reflecting team again, the family agreed that father may have had reservations about his wife going to work. However, he said that he would never stand in her way and had "resigned" himself to her returning. They also thought that it would be best to focus on the problem with which they were all concerned and which they were presenting to us: they had different expectations of Kim and related to her in very different ways.

At the end of the session the team suggested a variation of an "odd days/even days" ritual (Selvini-Palazzoli, Boscolo, Cecchin & Prata, 1978). The week was divided into three-day slots. On day one the family would treat Kim as an older daughter, like mother would want her to be; on day two they would treat her like a younger child as her father wanted; and on day three there were no set arrangements as to how to relate to Kim or how she should act. All liked the idea and Kim agreed to follow her parents' request on each day and act accordingly.

When the family came for its next meeting, they reported that they had done the ritual for the first few days and then stopped. Kim stated that she liked doing it a lot. Being with her parents was easier with their expectations clarified for her. However, on "younger days" she missed having the kind of conversations that she had had with her mother when she was treated as an "equal." On "older days" she missed the kind of contact that she had with her brother and sister and the attention that she received from her father. Mr. and Mrs. Hunter started to talk more with one another and less through Kim. At home they "spontaneously" began to discuss the possibility of Mrs. Hunter going back to work and decided on a date.

Mr. Hunter realized that he had been trying to keep his "baby" a little girl, while Mrs. Hunter felt that she was placing Kim in a too adult role, as she had been placed when she was a child. They talked about what aspects of each other's behaviors they liked, wanted to keep and what they wanted to change.

There were two more therapy sessions to continue the discussion that they had been having at home, and the parents were seen once without the children to discuss the issue concerning Mrs. Hunter's desire to work. During the remainder of the summer Kim became closer to her sister and spent a great deal of time with her.

During the course of therapy there was some brief discussion of Mike's hurling "accident" in the office and all reported that he had been doing very well at home and at school with no other incidents. No one saw him as problematic and there was no further discussion about the incident.

During a follow-up a year later, Mrs. Hunter had been working full time, 3:00 to 11:00 p.m., and Mr. Hunter had been taking care of the three kids while she was at work. All was still going well. Therapy lasted a total of six sessions.

Discussion

In this case, like the one above, the child helped highlight a previously undiscussed, undisclosed issue. There are numerous explanations for Mike's response in this situation. The primary issue for this discussion is that as one result of his behavior his parents were able to view their situation differently. Perhaps he was experiencing a tremendous loyalty bind, "knowing" that he could not speak up for his mother, being so close to his father, but feeling that he must act in some way. Perhaps there was some idea that a drastic step was needed to move the family into the next stage of their transition. Families follow a natural progression of transitions along the family life-cycle, but they were stalled. They were responding to the situation with ways that had been useful at a former stage of family development, but which were no longer applicable. Through the course of therapy they were able to move out of their stuck positions regarding themselves and the children and make the transition as a family into the next developmental stage of the family life-cycle. (For a further description and explanation of the family life-cycle, see Gordetsky & Zilbach, 1989, pp. 95-115; Zilbach, 1988).

The team provided a non-blaming perspective with a variety of ideas which the family could accept or not. The team tried to represent all positions that they were able to see within the family, not taking any side, but keeping to a both/and position. A logical connotation for their behavior was offered to the family and that, coupled with the ritual, allowed them to make a shift in their view and in their behavior. They were able to develop a new solution that contained aspects of both parents' views as well as begin to address old personal issues of their own.

The Boy Who Instructs the Team

Mrs. Page called regarding her eight-year-old son, Paul, who was afraid that the "sun would get too hot and fall out of the sky," had stomach aches, and feared going on plane trips. The family consisted of mother, 31, father, 33, Paul, 8, and a younger daughter, Sandy, 5. All were asked to come to the first meeting. In the initial interview Mrs. Page said that coming for a consultation was her idea and that she was the most concerned about the situation. She had first thought of coming four months ago, but her husband thought that "the situation might straighten itself out on its own." She reported that she had seen a psychiatrist for a year and a half for depression and that seeing her son "go through this" reminded her of herself. Mr. Page said that he was not opposed to this meeting, but tended to procrastinate and probably would not have come if it were up to him.

When Mrs. Page listed her concerns about Paul, he disqualified each one, saying that they were "only that one time" or "that was because of . . . ," etc. Sandy sat on her mother's lap during this with Paul sitting next to mother on the couch. Mr. Page sat alone in a chair. Mrs. Page agreed that these problems do not occur "all the time," but they "stick with her" long after they are over: she feels bad when they happen, questions herself whether she has "accomplished anything as a mother," feels a lowering of her self-confidence, and is reminded of "what I went through" as a child. When asked if others knew what she went through, she said that only her sister knew. She reported that she was one of twelve children and was only close to this one sister who had the same experiences that she did.

As Mrs. Page said this, she became tearful and Paul moved over to sit on her lap as Sandy moved off. Mrs. Page continued, saying that if Paul did not have these problems her concerns hopefully would get "buried deeper and deeper," and she would not think about them. She found this "forgetting" more desirable than constantly being reminded of them. If she did not have these memories she would have the same attitude toward Paul's difficulties that her husband held.

The interview moved very slowly. Mr. Page offered only one-line responses and deferred to his wife for any information about the children, saying that she "knew about these things as she had raised them so far." He said that he was the youngest of six children and had a very stable childhood. He had no understanding of what his wife could be remembering, as they had never discussed it. He said that he would like to get help for her so that she could "stand all this better."

At this point the therapist and family switched places with the reflecting team. The team initially commented on the pace of the interview, which they sensed showed a great deal of care and concern for all family members by one another. They noted how sensitive each of the children seemed to be toward each parent and how the therapist moved very carefully through the interview. One team member was curious when Mrs. Page first might have been feeling depressed or begun thinking about these old memories: did this occur before or after her son's problems were noticed and did they think the two problems were connected in any way? Does her son also believe that she would feel better if the problems were buried deeper? A question was raised whether these memories should be discussed or not. Were these memories perhaps too painful to be discussed and best left dormant? Another member wondered if these memories were discussed, who should be present? Might Mrs. Page discuss them alone with the therapist or with her husband present? Would he want to be present? Should the children be present or not?

The therapist and family switched places again with the reflecting team and *both* children immediately sat on mother's lap. She agreed that they were sensitive children and knew both parents well. She then agreed that these memories could be talked about, without the children there, but with her husband present. Mr. Page agreed.

At that moment, both children got up and went to the toy area and started to play. This was the first time they had left their mother's side during the entire interview. When asked what they thought about the team's comments, Paul said he disagreed with everything: "They should have said 'case closed!'"

Discussion

The children's non-verbal response to the reflections by the team were taken as a very strong message: this was not their issue, but their mother's and father's. This was not something that they could have verbalized. As in the Hunter family above, the boy's relationship with his father may have been very deep: he could not have verbalized his concern that his or his mother's problems may have been serious without betraying the loyalty binds that he believed he had with his father. He could only express these concerns through non-verbal actions, guiding the therapist in a direction which could be taken.

The relationship between Paul's fears and his mother's issues was yet to be seen and there was the question whether his fears would subside in the near future or not. These concerns could be monitored in therapy through his mother, and he could be invited back to a future session.

Mirroring aspects of reflections were demonstrated by the team's comments on the family's and therapist's verbal and non-verbal behaviors in the interview and through their use of a subdued tone, slow pace and the specific language of different family members. In addition, the reflections included speculations through the introduction of questions that were not raised during the meeting.

This last issue is particularly important in the model and in this interview. Often a therapist may feel that she/he is not able to ask certain questions, for whatever reasons, particularly in cases where there is violence, suspected incest, alcohol/substance abuse, etc. Sometimes the therapist is unable to think of any other questions to ask. Whatever the reason, the therapist's behavior is viewed in its contextual relationship at that moment and should be respected. The team, in its reflections, is able to introduce different thoughts and questions which the therapist did not or could not, allowing the therapist to continue in the conversation with the family without being viewed as attached to these potentially too different issues. This process allows the therapist to continue to maintain a neutral position and possibly explore these other issues with the family system as a participant in the conversation.

In the case above the therapist felt that he had to tread very carefully, given the tentativeness of the father and the continued disqualifications by the son. The therapist had to stay very close to what the family was willing to discuss and to the actions of the young children. This was done by not asking questions that may have been too "hard" or unusual for the family or pressing treatment on them. The team was able to introduce several ideas, very tentatively, that the family was able to accept. The family was then able to provide both the therapist and the team with the necessary feedback, verbally and non-verbally, regarding the correctness of these ideas for this system and to continue in treatment.

SUMMARY

These cases demonstrate how the inclusion of young children in family therapy greatly increases the range in which the therapist can work. The reflecting team model offers a respectful and useful framework for their inclusion. Children can provide the team and the family with valuable "information" or "news of a difference" both during the interview and in response to the team's reflections.

To limit children's participation when they are clearly a part of the problem system is to limit the family's and the therapist's abilities to generate new distinctions and help foster change. With the strong theoretical emphasis of the reflecting team model on constructivism and that all views may be potentially useful ones, it seems particularly appropriate to utilize this model with families with young children. It is often these small "voices" that need to be recognized and listened to.

NOTE

1. The switches that take place during the interview may be done in a variety of ways. With the team sitting in an observation room, the lights and sound between the two rooms may be switched, allowing the family and therapist to watch and listen to the team make its comments. The therapist and family also may switch places with the team, going behind the mirror and having the team come into the consulting room. In the absence of a mirror, the team may be in the room with the client system, maintaining an imaginary boundary between themselves and the clients. With only two therapists both may wish to be in the room, having one remain silent during the interview and then "reflect" with the interviewer.

REFERENCES

Andersen, T. (1987). The reflecting team: Dialogue and meta-dialogue in clinical work. *Family Process, 26*(4), 415-428.
Andersen, H., Goolishian, H. and Winderman, L. (1986). Problem determined systems: Towards transformation in family therapy. *Journal of Strategic and Systemic Therapies, 5*(4), 1-11.
Bateson, G. (1972). *Steps to an ecology of mind.* New York: Ballantine Books.
Bloch, D. (1976). Including the children in family therapy. In P. Guerin (Ed.), *Family therapy: Theory and practice.* New York: Gardner Press.
Bogdan, J. (1984). Family organization as an ecology of ideas. *Family Process, 23*, 375-388.
Boscolo, L., Cecchin, G., Hoffman, L. and Penn, P. (1987). *Milan systemic family therapy.* New York: Basic Books.
Carter, B. and McGoldrick, M. (1980). *The family life cycle: A framework for family therapy.* New York: Gardner Press.
Combrinck-Graham, L. (1986). *Treating young children in family therapy.* Maryland: Aspen Press.
Dowling, E. and Jones, H. V. R. (1978). Small children seen and heard in family therapy. *Journal of Child Psychiatry, 4*(4), 87-96.
von Foerster, H. (1981). *Observing systems.* Seaside, CA: Intersystems Publication.

von Glasersfeld, E. (1984). An introduction to radical constructivism. In P. Watzlawick (Ed.), *The invented reality*. New York: W. W. Norton.

Haley, J. (1973). *Uncommon therapy: The psychiatric techniques of Milton Erickson, M.D.*, New York: W. W. Norton.

Hoffman, L. (1986). Beyond power and control. *Family Systems Medicine, 3*, 381-396.

Hoffman, L. (March, 1987). Family therapy as a science of compassion. *Tenth Family Therapy Network Conference*, Washington, DC.

Imber-Coppersmith, E. (1985). Families and multiple helpers: A systemic perspective. In D. Campbell and R. Draper (Eds.), *Applications of systemic family therapy: The Milan approach*. London: Academic Press.

MacKinnon, L. and Miller, D. (1987). The new epistemology and the Milan approach: Feminist and sociopolitical considerations. *Journal of Marriage and Family Therapy, 13*(2), 139-156.

Maloney, M. (1981). The use of children's drawings in multiple family group therapy. *Group, 5*(4), 32-36.

Maturana, H. (November, 1984). Plenary speech. *Annual Meeting of the American Society for Cybernetics*, Philadelphia, PA.

Neisser, U. (1976). *Cognition and reality*. San Francisco: Freeman.

Penn, P. (1982). Circular questioning. *Family Process, 21*, 267-280.

Penn, P. (1985). Feed-forward: Future questions, future maps. *Family Process, 24*, 299-311.

Powers, W. (1973). *Behavior: The control of perception*. Chicago: Aldine.

Selvini-Palazzoli, M., Boscolo, L., Cecchin, G. and Prata, G. (1980). Hypothesizing-circularity-neutrality: Three guidelines for the conductor of the session. *Family Process, 19*, 3-12.

Selvini-Palazzoli, M., Boscolo, L., Cecchin, G. and Prata, G. (1978). A ritualized prescription in family therapy: Odd days and even days. *Journal of Marriage and Family Counseling*, July.

Steier, F. and Smith, K. K. (1985). Organizations and second order cybernetics. *Journal of Strategic and Systemic Therapies, 4*(4), 53-65.

Tomm, K. (1985). Circular interviewing: A multifaceted clinical tool. In D. Campbell and R. Draper (Eds.), *Applications of systemic family therapy: The Milan approach*. London: Academic Press.

Verheij, F. (1980). The child and family therapy. *Acta Paedopsychiatrica, 46*(3), 161-174.

Weiner, N. (1961). *Cybernetics*. (2nd ed.). Cambridge: MIT Press.

Wolfe, L. and Collins, J. (1983). Action techniques for therapy with families with young children. *Family Relations, 32*(1), 81-87.

Zilbach, J. J. (1974). The family in family therapy. *Journal of the American Academy of Child Psychiatry, 13*(3), 459-467.

Zilbach, J. J. (1986). *Young children in family therapy*. New York: Brunner/Mazel.

Zilbach, J. J. (1988). The family life cycle: A framework for understanding children in family therapy. In L. Combrinck-Graham (Ed.), *Children in Family Contexts*. New York: Guilford Press.

Zilbach, J. J., Bergel, E. W. and Gass, C. (1968). The family life cycle: Some developmental considerations. Proceedings of the IVth International Congress of Group Psychotherapy. *Verlag der Weiner Medizinischen Akademie*, Vienna, 157-162.

Zilbach, J. J., Bergel, E. N. and Gass, C. (1972). The role of the young child in family therapy. In C. J. Sager and H. S. Kaplan (Eds.), *Progress in group and family therapy*. New York: Brunner/Mazel.

Young Children and Play
in Object Relations
Family Therapy

David E. Scharff

Object relations family therapy is built upon the supposition that the inner life of individuals can often best be understood in the context of the family which contains and supports them.[1] Fairbairn's (1952) object relations theory of personality is built upon the premise that what primarily motivates each of us is the fundamental need for relationships. Our integral psychological structure is built up of the internalization of relationships, and the vicissitudes of individual development are the vicissitudes of the struggle to remain related and, at the same time, separate. Individuals need to feel held safely and securely by the broader family. This is true for the adults as well as for the children, although in different ways. As holding is established, more focused relationships thrive, offering vehicles for conscious and unconscious communication.

For families with young children, the children's play is the vehicle of communication between children and other family members for the issues around focused relating — the expression of internal object relations. But the play also communicates the quality of the family's capacity to supply holding for each other. It does so through the presence or absence of the children's capacity to play, through sibling interaction and parental management during play, and through themes about holding.

David E. Scharff, MD, is Director, The Washington School of Psychiatry.

[1]Scharff, D.E. and Scharff, J.S. (1987). *Object Relations Family Therapy*. Northvale, NJ: Jason Aronson.

The family therapist learns a great deal by attending to play in family sessions—to its expression of themes which pertain to the individual child and to the family as a whole. It is not, however, necessary to be fully trained in play therapy technique to do so. As the therapist attending to the themes the child is expressing, translating the play into a verbal narrative for himself or herself, the therapist can begin to make sense of the play. But the most important messages about the family are taken in through the absorption of family transference. This is partly a cognitive matter—a "decoding" of verbal and play messages the family gives. But a crucial part of understanding the family occurs through the therapist's countertransference, by close attention to the feelings and momentary identifications stirred up by the family in the course of a session and over time. The countertransference response then needs to be understood and fed back to the family, either in words or sometimes using the play.

The following session presents an example of a family in the mid-phase of treatment. It illustrates the use of play and how the interface between the family and therapist can be understood through the therapist's countertransference.

The Simpson family had been in treatment for about a year. They had come initially because of sexual difficulty between the parents: Mrs. S said that she "hated sex" while Mr. S had premature ejaculation. In addition, she was recurrently depressed while Mr. S had so much trouble with his memory that it interfered with his work as a computer programmer. They had readily agreed to a family evaluation because of difficulty with their middle child, a five-year-old boy, Alex, who soiled and wet his pants and was broadly immature. In that evaluation, I had felt that the 3 1/2-year-old girl, Jeanette, was also immature and over-excited, perhaps over-sexualized or seductive, and that the oldest, Eric, was a boy with solid latency development. However, in re-evaluation a year later, I saw the internalization of Eric's aggression too. He used a Superman action figure to attack Jeanette's helpless baby dolls and proclaimed that Superman had become an evil force. I had not seen Eric's internalized aggression earlier. The parents, however, were now in better shape: a year's intensive psychotherapy with a colleague had allowed Mrs. S to flourish. She was less frequently depressed, although she still had severe regressions and had been hospitalized for a few days in April. She had taken and maintained a part-time job and she was now interested in sex. The couple still needed sex therapy, but it looked as though the first priority was family work.

The session I will report came after approximately eight months of weekly family work. We had not been able to meet the previous week, but in the session two weeks earlier, I had investigated the central role of the mother's depression in the family and had been able to understand with them the role of each of the other family members in relation to it. Today, two weeks after that session, they came in, the children leading eagerly as usual. Eric began by showing me pictures of transformer robots he had drawn. These were called "Demolishicons," the most powerful of which was "Demolishicor." He then began to build with the collection of colored blocks which all three of them liked to use. Alex began to draw. Father suggested he draw Donald Duck. When he said he could not, Father said "He can *be* Donald Duck, but he can't draw it." Alex drew a Mickey Mouse face while Jeanette ate candy from a packet. They were all whispering.

I asked about the candy and the whispering. Was there a secret which led to the whispering?

They said there was no secret. They had arrived a half hour early and Mother got the candy because her mouth was dry from antidepressant medication. The side effects of blurred vision and dry mouth were not nearly so bad as at first. The discussion of her medication brought into the room memories of her recent hospitalization and the panic she had felt which led to it. As she talked, A handed her a second picture he had been drawing of "Monstro the Whale," who A said had swallowed Gepetto, Pinocchio's puppet-maker father. J handed her mother a picture which she said was "the primary colors" and she named them for me.

So far I felt that the activity in the room was avoidant, although not unusually so for the opening part of a session which followed both the previously moving one and after a missed session.

The session proceeded. Eric was now building a small building which he said was a museum. It was the same sort of structure he had built the last time, and he told me, the same sort of thing was going on there. "Nothing!" Eric wanted more cars and blocks to complete his design, which meant A should surrender some of his. Father and A tried to help him think how he might do so with what was available and without taking something from A.

Mother said, "Eric, if you can't have it the way you want, it would be nice to try to have it another way."

Eric rejected her advice and began to pout.

Noticing that the museum was loaded with toy soldiers with rifles with all the guns pointed straight at me, I said, "I see that all the guns are pointed right at me!" The family laughed. "Why am I the enemy? What bad thing am I about to do?" I asked.

Eric now took an action figure of the Incredible Hulk, a great green unfriendly looking figure and had it menace me playfully. It was coming to fight. I thought about the way the Hulk had often provided an analogy for anger in the family. In a session some months previously, we had talked about the way Mother felt she was an uncontrollable Hulk who wreaked damage on the family when she meant to work for the good. I now searched for a toy with which to engage the Hulk in dialogue.

Mother handed me a baby doll, saying "Babies have been known to be vicious."

I felt her offer indicated her identification with me as the object of Eric's anger, so I handed the doll back to her and said, "Maybe the baby can find out what I've done wrong."

She obligingly took the baby and through it said to the Hulk, "OK, Hulk, What have I done?"

Eric said for the Hulk, "I'm mad because you won't let me rule."

Mother said, "You can't always have your way and pinching won't help." The doll and the Hulk wrestled.

A interjected, "The baby lost her diaper and she's going to poop all over the floor." He stepped in to fight playfully with the Hulk himself. We were all aware that A's encopresis had now entered the discussion about anger.

I said, "A said that when the Hulk attacked the baby, she would lose control of her poops. Can people control their poops when they fight?"

A minute later A stopped the fight and took a car with which he knocked over the museum Eric had built.

Eric got angry, saying "Alex! Why did you have to do that?" He dropped the Hulk and began to rebuild the museum.

I said, "When A got between the Hulk and the baby, he talked about people losing control of their poops. But instead of losing control of his own poops like a baby this time, he destroyed the museum and Eric got mad. How does this relate to family events?"

Mother said, "Eric acts aggressive, but if you return it in kind, he doesn't like it. He thinks his own actions are OK, but in others they're wrong."

I said, lightly touching Eric's shoulder to get his attention, and I think, because I felt this discussion would be hard for him, "So you're saying, Mom, that Eric expects that he can play like the Hulk without objection. And he's surprised if someone else gets mad."

Eric asks me not to touch him on the shoulder. He has a sunburn. But I realize that he is not experiencing what I'm saying as sympathetic, and he'd like me to "lay off." He has been rebuilding the museum, and A now puts a family of small dolls in a car and drives over to visit the museum. I realize that A is not now acting like a soiling baby — a stance he has used so often — but is playing out the aggressive problem in an age-appropriate way. Eric has Demolishicor attack A's family.

Father says, "Jeanette and A can't stop Eric. He ignores it when they try to defend themselves, and he overwhelms them."

Mother had now turned red, and she spat out, "I'm livid. When he does this, I get so mad. Right now, I just want to leave the room!"

I said, "Tell me about it instead."

She said, "I can't discuss my anger yet. I feel he's so stubborn, even after you point it out to him. It causes everyone else to be unhappy. He monopolizes things like the blocks. I just want to knock over that museum."

I turned to Eric, with whom I was now feeling identified, and said, "Eric, does this happen at home?"

Nodding slowly with tears in his eyes, he acknowledged it did.

Father said, "Usually things break down at this point. Eric, give some of the blocks to A and Jeanette."

Mother said, "Eventually we intervene. Then he's upset we have forced his hand."

Father said, "Then Eric feels we favor A and Jeanette."

"Is that right?" I asked Eric.

He nodded sorrowfully, putting his head down on a table and becoming inert.

"What is this like from your growing up, Mrs. S?" I asked.

"It's like my father," she said. "We would dread the time he came home when he would line us up and yell at us, looking for someone who did something wrong. Then if one of us admitted something, he would yell at that one. It was awful. He had to be in charge. He made the rules, and no one else mattered. And my mother didn't protect us from him. Just like I can't protect Jeanette and A."

"So you feel that Eric is like your father, whom you felt was so destructive?" I asked.

She nodded, beginning to sob. "And when I feel that and I get so mad at him, then I feel that I'm like my father too, and I hate that worse than anything in the world. I hated that man, and now I'm just like him. And then I hate Eric worse for making me feel that way."

Seeing Eric now slumping over the table, Father said to him, "come here, Son." Eric got up slowly and accepted a loving hug from his father, draped across his chest while Father stroked his arm and back. It looked terribly comforting, and at the same time, it did not get in the way of the work which was going on. I felt grateful to Father for comforting Eric in a way which let Mother keep speaking. He was managing to hold the family in holding Eric. It let me keep my attention on Mother. Jeanette now went to her and climbed in her lap, comforting her, and A continued to play with the remains of the museum, building a simpler building to house the car family he had been using.

I said to Mother, "When you feel you're bad like your own father, you hate Eric, but you also hate yourself."

"Yes," she sobbed. "And I feel I've damaged him just the way I felt my father hurt me. And I can't undo it. There isn't any way out."

It was excruciating in the room. I wondered what despair I had wrought. And at the same time, I felt almost exhilarated that the family was managing to hold a steady course through these straits of despair.

I wanted to enlarge the field of this moment to include Father, so I turned to him and asked, "Does this have any echoes for you, too?"

He said, "My childhood wasn't so dramatic. At least I don't remember any events like that. Sometimes we'd be spanked with a belt for doing something wrong. I can't remember anything more."

Thinking of Father's inability to remember so many things, I said, "Of course, you're not being able to remember is one of the things you struggle with. What would you be spanked for?"

"I only remember one time," he said. "I was spanked for going over to a little girlfriend's house when I was about Eric's age. My dad womped me with his belt. It hurt. I can relate to Eric's sulking now when I think about it."

I turned to Eric, "Did you know about your Dad's being spanked with a belt?" I asked. Eric shook his head.

Over the next couple of minutes, we established that in Father's recollection, what he had been punished for had a sexual connotation: he had been strapped at least partly because he had disappeared with a girl.

I now said, "Mrs. S, you get so mad at Eric because he reminds you of your father, then you feel like the bad parent yourself when you get so mad. He feels destructive and hopeless to get your love. Through all of this, Mr. S lives through you in a way, feeling that any sexual interest will invoke an angry father. The two of you have a similar struggle, Mr. and Mrs. S, when sexual matters are at issue. But in the setting with the children, it is often Eric who is in the role of bringing up the bad father. When he wants something for himself, he feels bad about it, and he becomes a Demolishicor. But he also does it in a way to keep you, Mrs. S, from feeling that you are the Hulk or the Demolishicor yourself."

Mother said, "Yes, you're right. And I want to bust up his museum because I don't want him to be so high and mighty. Then I feel awful." At this moment, A took the car and broke down the last remains of the museum.

I said, "And it is at those times that A takes on Eric for you, Mrs.

S. It is part of the reason A is so hard to stop in his impulsive destructiveness." He used to do it by becoming an angry, pooping baby. These days he is getting more directly angry.

Jeanette climbed down from her mother's lap and began to play sweetly among the ruins.

Father was rubbing Eric's head. I asked him, "What do you think is happening now?"

He said, "Eric's hurt. He has a hard time when his Mom is so unhappy with him. There are things he wants to do better and doesn't know how to change.

I asked Eric, "Is that right?"

He nodded.

Mother said, "He probably hates me back."

I said, "So you're afraid he'll hate you like you hate your father? But is there anything else you feel for Eric?"

"Oh, yes! I love him. Really I do. He's a wonderful kid. I don't know what else. I feel hopeless, like all the damage is done. He's already been hurt. I've done it. I hate myself." And she begins to sob again.

A begins now to build a simpler house from the blocks, one to house the family car.

I said to Eric, "Do you still feel like crying?"

"Yes," he said. "I feel sad."

"I know you do," I said.

> And I think this has been painful for everyone, your Mom included. But it's important we talk about all this because it's underneath so much of what goes wrong at home. It gets in the way of the loving. In your family, Mrs. S, you felt your Dad hated you and you hated him, but you wanted his love. What's so painful about being so mad at Eric is how much you care about him too, and feel for him being in a situation like yours. And you also envy him being so competent, getting so much, and then wanting more. It makes you remember how you've felt you have so little. This image of the bad father comes out at these moments of breakdown. It often keeps you, Mr. and Mrs. S, from feeling you can be good parents. Each of you has felt that you couldn't get enough love now or when you were

little, so now there isn't enough to go around. It gets played out in the way we've seen. If someone wants too much, it's as though he is taking it from the rest of the family. And finally, I think this may also be operating in the sexual relationship, at least from the clue Mr. S's memory gives us. But that we'll have to explore with the two of you alone. What's important today is the way each of you plays out the anger over what's missing, and the painful effects when it goes wrong. We have to have these moments in the family therapy—despite the pain—or we can't learn this kind of thing.

This example illustrates the use of play in a mid-phase session where interpretive work is possible. Family and therapist share an understanding of the children's play and of their interaction while they play and talk. The children play while they listen, understand the allusions that their parents and the therapist make to the meaning of their play. Through the session, a shared understanding of the current version of the family's dilemma grows.

This happens as individual contributions to the theme coalesce in the experience of the family and the therapist. The countertransference reflected my vacillating identifications—with the oldest boy, with the parents as they handled sibling bickering, with the encopretic boy, and finally with the overall family as they struggled to manage the problems in providing holding to each other and to themselves as a group. At the end I was able to formulate an understanding of the family group as a whole as it struggled with the vicissitudes of individual needs and relationships and with the difficulty of balancing one person's needs for love and understanding with those of others. This is the work of object relations family therapy. The understanding and use of play, the full integration of the needs and contributions of young children, and the availability of the therapist to make sense of inner experience all contribute to this shared venture.

Countertransference in Psychodynamic Family Therapy with Children

Susan Scholfield-MacNab

The field that you are standing before appears to have the same proportions as your own life.

John Berger
About Looking

Emotions are the responses that link our inner and outer worlds. Countertransference is rooted in our emotions and often manifests itself in the form of affective experiences. Each new situation that we encounter is colored by affective associations to important earlier relationships. Countertransference is often portrayed as a negative phenomenon in which these emotional associations to past relationships interfere with the present therapeutic relationship.

But countertransference responses can offer the family therapist more than distorted perceptions. Countertransference is also the primary source of our empathic understanding of the families with whom we work. Our therapeutic interventions are guided, in part, by our affective responses to the complex interweaving of past with present; and our associations to personal experiences stirred by material from patient families. These experiences are all part of a professionally trained clinical perspective. To disavow or exclude the data provided by our countertransferential responses, is to unnecessarily limit the tools available to us in the difficult task of listening to and making meaning of communications from families.

Countertransference is defined as the whole of the therapist's re-

Susan Scholfield-MacNab, PhD, is affiliated with the Boston Institute of Psychotherapies.

sponses to the stimulus presented by the patient family. These responses are due to the evocation of some part of the therapist's own personal history or present life situations, or to her reaction to the powerful affect of the patient family (independent of her own history), or all of the above (MacNab, 1987, p. 102). Powerful affective states within the family system are transmitted verbally and non-verbally, and the therapist can observe her own emotional resonances to some or all of these transmissions.

> The signals from the family's struggle, by necessity, get mixed up with the therapist's own similar struggles . . . the therapist invokes memories of personal work with similar struggles as a way of making the whole process more available consciously, working toward a reunderstanding of the issues. Of course, some issues will have been more conflictual for the therapist than others. (Scharff, D. & Scharff, J., 1987, p. 225)

In family therapy, the therapist meets with children and adults — the ages can range from infancy to old age. Attention to countertransference phenomena provides the therapist with information that can aid the search for answers to important clinical questions. How does the therapist understand her many reactions to such a varied group, including children who communicate with drawings or other forms of play rather than words? How does she categorize and find the meaning in the often highly evocative play of the children in the family? The relationship between an adult (the therapist) and a child reflects the different developmental capabilities of each of them. Do these differences evoke compassionate or discomforting responses? How can the therapist organize the myriad associations from her professional knowledge about child and family development, from her own childhood experiences and from her own present life circumstances to find the true nature of the message the family is sending? How does the therapist sort out these complexities as she struggles to listen and to understand the whole family system? What are the intrapsychic, the interpersonal and the sociocultural components of the emotional reactions and at what level of consciousness do they occur?

Because there are so many sources of countertransference responses to families with children, the therapist needs to organize the various dimensions of communications involved in her responses to them. The following statement from *Young Children in Family Therapy* refers to some of these important countertransference responses:

> Finally, as adults, therapists have had to renounce, in the course of their own development, the world of their childhood with varying degrees of reluctance; the danger to adult therapists of having childhood feelings and issues rearoused by including young children in family therapy is not to be discounted. (Zilbach, 1986, p. 76)

A comprehensive model of countertransference in psychodynamic family therapy will include the following dimensions: intrapsychic, interpersonal and sociocultural phenomena; from three time periods, the therapist's childhood (family of origin), her present life circumstances ranging from her familial relationships to her professional training, and the therapy session itself with the accompanying boundary issues (such as fees, scheduling, confidentiality); the level of consciousness at which these responses from various aspects of her life are being evoked, i.e., conscious, preconscious and unconscious.

It is through examining countertransference that the therapist's responses can be fashioned into a useful tool for understanding and containing the troubled and troubling aspects of the family system. Her responses to the children in the family allow her to empathize with them, to understand their experience of their parents as a counterreaction to parents' experiences with them. The therapist's countertransferential responses provide the groundwork for an understanding of each member in the family and of the family as a whole. To ignore countertransference, an omnipresent element in all therapeutic encounters, is to risk abandoning the search for the meanings of intricately constructed family communications.

Countertransference in family therapy with children is a response to a particularly broad range of stimuli. For example, the behaviors of an identified child patient may require a delving into conscious and unconscious countertransferential responses in order to truly understand the family's experiences with this child.

> The diagnostic interview with the Morgan family began an hour after the family arrived because of scheduling confusion — either theirs or the clinic's secretary. Martha, 8, the oldest of two adopted children was being evaluated in a local mental health clinic following a school referral. The Morgans were a highly educated, well-known local family. During this initial interview Martha broke the therapist's desk stapler, ran around the office when asked a question by the therapist and eluded all of the therapist's attempts to verbally engage her. Meanwhile the parents and younger brother, 6, sat quietly together on the office sofa.

The therapist noticed that she was embarrassed by her difficulty in talking to the child, and that (unlike other interviews with hyperactive children) she could not focus on the meaning of the child's behavior or on engaging the entire family system during this initial interview. After the session she recalled a childhood incident in which she as a young child was reprimanded at a Christmas dinner in front of family friends for not taking care of her younger brother whose increasingly disruptive behavior was angering her mother and father. The countertransference embarrassment around public scoldings and strong family wishes for more controlled behavior had apparently been evoked by the constellation of this family. This memory helped her understand the meaning of Martha's behavior in this family. It was the markedly contrasting behaviors in the Morgan children, and the anger, embarrassment and helplessness represented by her own countertransference response to Martha's behavior that were the important clues to this family's dilemma. In addition, the public nature of this family's meetings with school personnel and a long period in the clinic's busy waiting room contained sociocultural issues (was it the family or the therapist, or both, who felt anxiety about upper-middle-class clients being seen in a clinic that traditionally served working-class and lower-class clients?) and therapy session boundary issues (such as confidentiality and scheduling consistency). Each of these incidents evoked a discomforting countertransferential response in the therapist, initially identifiable as due to her own professional concerns about the boundaries around the therapy, and an apologetic awkwardness evoked by the family's exposure to the chaos in the waiting room where they were seated with a number of welfare clients. These were countertransferential responses that informed the therapist of the need to examine both her potential over-identification with the family's emphasis on status, and her realistic professional concerns.

Without this kind of exploration of countertransferential responses, linked with a conceptual understanding of countertransference issues, the therapist would have been less able to identify and to break out of the projections of the family. The therapist's willingness to sort out her own family of origin issues, her present family life experiences, and her professional concerns as honestly as possible, coupled with her affectual experiences, set the stage for therapeutic change. These are not experiences that therapists regularly discuss directly with families, for example in this case the therapist decided that her own heightened awareness of these issues would be sufficient to help her listen more clearly to the family's concerns. The therapist's ability to understand her countertransference reactions to children; using such tools as associations, memories, self-knowledge, and supervision can increase her empathy and understanding of the whole family and their struggles.

The communication between therapist and family, and the therapist's countertransference responses include an aspect of projective identification. Projective identification is an intrapsychic and interpersonal phenomenon in which the projector unconsciously imagines that one unwanted aspect of himself is now part of another person. The projector then pressures the recipient of the projections to act as if he now contains that aspect within himself. The recipient then processes the projections in accord with his own character and acts in accord with the behaviors and feelings of the projected material. The degree to which the recipient transforms the projected material depends on the intactness of the ego boundaries of the recipient, and the nature of the relationship between projector and recipient. In psychodynamic family therapy, the therapist allows herself to become the recipient of the family's projections, and then to contain the projections and translate them into more modulated secondary processes which she helps the family reinternalize. These aspects of themselves are then experienced in a more conscious, accepting and mature manner. It is this process of the therapist identifying and accepting the projections of unwanted aspects of the family's experiences that is a difficult, but essential part of the therapeutic process. To be able to diagnose the source of an unexpected response requires an understanding of the family's history, one's own history and the conscious and unconscious interplay between the two. Ogden describes projective identification in this way:

> . . . the projector [in his case the patient family members] has the primarily unconscious fantasy of ridding himself of unwanted aspects of the self: depositing those unwanted parts in another person; and finally, recovering a modified version of what was extruded. (Ogden, 1982, p. 11)

The exploration of these particularly complex psychological phenomena is a central feature of a therapeutic understanding of the family's troubles. Projective identification occurs between family members as well as between family members and the therapist. Among the motivations for collusion between children and parents in this process can be the child's

> . . . fear of object loss which might ensue were he not to act in behalf of the parent's defensive organisation . . . [the child is] walking a fine line between fulfillment of their own strivings for an autonomous identity and conformity with . . . a parental defense. (Zinner, J. & Shapiro, R., 1972, p. 12)

Observing these collusions between parents and children, and the anxiety they are designed to ward off also leads the therapist to an exploration of countertransference responses. It can be a highly charged experience to witness the pain involved in projective identifications between parents and children. The ability to tolerate and explore these interactions is essential to the containment, transformation, and reintrojection of projective identifications which are an important curative factor in psychodynamic family therapy.

In all psychotherapy modalities the unconscious reactions are the most difficult for the therapist to identify and to bring into consciousness. Families bring an especially powerful communal energy to bear on the creation of transference states and resistances to therapeutic interventions. The patient family, coming into therapy with their chosen solutions to the difficulties they are facing, add their resistance to the therapist's own defensive reactions to the material. It is necessary for the therapist to undertake an analysis of all the elements, conscious, preconscious and unconscious of the communications between herself and the family.

Following several months of progress in play therapy with a withdrawn and seriously learning disabled young girl, Sherry, 6, the therapist began family therapy sessions. This was initiated by the therapist because of the mother's seeming reluctance to acknowledge her daughter's progress to such an extent that she was considering placing her in a residential program in another state. Prior to the first family meeting the therapist was quite anxious; she had some awareness that this was due to her attachment to the child (the therapist had a similar although less serious disability as the child) and her belief that the child should not be in a residential program. In the first family meeting the mother did not speak to the child, only to the therapist. With the therapist's encouragement, the mother gradually spoke with more affect about the disappointment this child had been to her. She suddenly said, "I sometimes hate her." The therapist quickly looked to see if the child had understood her mother, it was unclear and therefore the therapist decided to help the mother and daughter with this denied affect by asking the daughter to say what she heard and then having the mother verify it to her daughter. The therapist trembled throughout the entire interview. However, the working through of these feelings in subsequent family meetings led to increased attachment between Sherry and her mother and then the rest of the family. Her progress continued, with the mother becoming much more involved with her treatment and there was no further talk of institutionalization.

In this instance, the therapist's courage in following the mother's affect was made more possible through her understanding of her own identification with Sherry, and her strongly held negative beliefs about institutionalization. She sensed the similarity between her own mother's and Sherry's mother's anxiety about revealing the unconscious anger and disappointment about their daughters' disabilities. The acknowledgement of the therapist's and the mother's concerns was central to resolving the therapeutic impasse. The family was able to make a commitment to this child only after they worked through the previously unexpressed feelings about Sherry's problems. This process began with the therapist's attention to her own countertransferential responses, including her personal and professional beliefs and values about the placement of children outside of the home.

Identification with the child, or children, in family therapy is a major source of countertransference. The wish to protect the child and oneself from the pain of a troubled family is often overwhelming. It can lead to a change in modalities, i.e., deciding prematurely that a family is not sufficiently motivated for family work; excluding children from the actual session; or, as almost occurred in the above example, avoiding the real emotional work of the sessions. In this case the therapist began to see how upsetting it was to think of the rejection she imagined Sherry would feel if her mother went ahead with a plan to send her to a residential program. The therapist recalled the ways that her mother had rejected her, often through denial of her disability, and the unacknowledged fear and rage the denial represented. The anger that Sherry's mother expressed had parallels to the anger in the therapist's family and the subsequent wish to reject and deny this painful affect. This understanding reduced the therapist's anxiety and helped her support more open expression of previously unacceptable feelings in this family. The mother's first step toward resolving her ambivalence about keeping her child at home was voicing her feelings of frustration and hatred, first to the therapist and then to the child. From that session on the mother began to work with the realities of her child's problems.

In summary, the identification of the sources of countertransference responses involves an analysis of three dimensions: (1) Time—the therapist's childhood and adult experiences (including her professional training) and the here and now of the therapy setting; (2) Locus of Communication—her intrapsychic, interpersonal and sociocultural responses; and (3) Level of Consciousness—unconscious, preconscious and consciousness. These three dimensions describe the range of psychological phenomena that can be involved in countertransferential responses in family therapy. They each contain elements that can be evoked by work with families with children. This tripartite model provides a means of organizing the whole of the therapist's responses and identifying those of significance. The three dimensions of countertransference phenomena can be described as follows:

(1) This dimension describes which temporal aspects of the therapist's experience are being evoked. Are the responses more directly related to current professional issues or to childhood experiences? For example, is the move from child therapy to family therapy in the second example sufficiently supported by the therapist's training and education so that she is confident about her clinical decision and her abilities as a family therapist? Is the work setting supportive of the modality of family therapy? Or, are the experiences being evoked located in the therapist's more distant past, in her family of origin? This is the most frequently discussed source of countertransference, often presented as a difficulty to be cleared away. While it is no doubt true that family of origin experiences can be sufficiently troubling so that they repeatedly interfere with therapist's ability to help families with certain kinds of problems, if these memories can be made conscious and tolerated (either alone or with supervision and/or therapy) they are also a rich source of understanding for families in treatment.

(2) The inner and outer worlds of the therapist can be located along a continuum of intrapsychic, interpersonal and sociocultural beliefs and values. For example, the class issues evoked by vignette of the Morgan family may, in addition to identifying the therapist's own experiences and values, also highlight family's current difficulties.

(3) The level of consciousness at which the countertransferential responses occur is crucial to a thorough exploration of countertransference, and particularly crucial to the resolution of projective identifications. If the therapist can creatively explore the clues contained in her anxieties and fantasies, and note how much repression is evoked in her by this material, the unconscious meanings of her

responses can be used to increase her ability to listen to the family and to understand why she has these reactions to certain of their communications.

Each of these three dimensions forms a continuum: from the remote past to the here and now; from intrapsychic to sociocultural; and from unconscious to conscious. An understanding of where on each continuum countertransferential responses occur helps the therapist to welcome children's delightfully creative communications into the family's therapy.

REFERENCES

MacNab, S. (1987). Countertransference in Psychodynamic Family Therapy. Unpublished doctoral dissertation, The Fielding Institute, Santa Barbara, CA.

Ogden, T. (1982). *Projective Identification and Psychotherapeutic Technique.* New York: Jason Aronson.

Scharff, D. & Scharff, J. (1987). *Object Relations Family Therapy.* Northvale, NJ: Jason Aronson.

Zilbach, J. (1986). *Young Children in Family Therapy.* New York, NY: Brunner/ Mazel.

Zinner, J. & Shapiro, R. (1972). Projective Identification As a Mode of Perception and Behavior in Families of Adolescents, *International Journal of Psychoanalysis, 53.*

Child and Family Therapy: An Integrated Approach

Sharon Gordetsky
Joan J. Zilbach

Every family has a specific family developmental history and family developmental process of its own which make up the Family Life Cycle which is separate from, although certainly influenced by, the developmental histories of the individual family members. Often a familial developmental impasse results in a child becoming "problematic," "difficult," or symptomatic. Therefore, it is essential to utilize both an individual and family developmental framework when we are evaluating and treating children and families. We ask what are the developmental issues and tasks that our individual child patient is attempting to master—intrapsychically and between him/herself and the environment; *and* what are the developmental issues and tasks for the family at this point in time. Finally, we must consider how they are likely to interact with each other, and the likely consequences for the family and individual child patient and other individual family members.

FAMILY DEVELOPMENT: THE FAMILY LIFE CYCLE

A chart of family development summarizes the Family Life Cycle, including the primary family stage markers, and core family

Sharon Gordetsky, PhD, is Chief Psychologist, Parents' and Children's Services, Boston, MA. Joan J. Zilbach, MD, is affiliated with the Fielding Institute, Santa Barbara, CA.

The authors want to thank Drs. Ruth Stern, Judith Reiner-Platt and David Bernstein for their help in reviewing this clinical material.

95

tasks (see Table A). Every family unit traverses this life cycle from beginning to end. (Revised from Zilbach, 1968, 1979, 1983, 1986.) The maintenance, continuity, expansion and even existence of every family is dependent upon specific basic family functions, some of which remain fairly constant throughout the family life cycle, and some that change according to the particular stage of family development.

There are two general categories of basic family functions: (1) those that enable a family to exist and enhance *intrafamilial* relationships and, (2) those that create bonds outside the family, with the community and the larger society, i.e., *extrafamilial* relationships.

The basic family functions include providing for: (1) intrafamilial: supplies/food, shelter/housing, finances/employment, health care; and (2) extrafamilial: adequate education, recreation, socialization and transmission of values.

We have found it extremely important and therapeutically useful to inquire about specific family functions in the presence of the entire family, requesting all family members to contribute to the discussion of these family functions. For example, asking the children to draw a picture of their house including their rooms or a picture of their family having dinner. Such a "simple" inquiry led to the discovery in one case that the family could not tolerate being together even for a meal. One of the children drew a picture of each family member eating his or her meal in a separate room doing a separate activity, i.e., the mother watched the soap opera she recorded daily on her VCR; the adolescent daughter ate while talking on the telephone in her room; the father read the newspaper; and the identified patient watched another TV show!

This paper will focus on the benefits of integrating ongoing family therapy sessions when there is an identified child patient in individual psychotherapy. Furthermore, it will address the contributions and benefits of including *all* family members (i.e., everyone living under the same roof), including the youngest children in family therapy. We will present and illustrate treatment strategies geared to enhance the active participation of children in family therapy sessions.

There are many reasons why the importance of family therapy

sessions are overlooked and undervalued, and/or when they do occur, that the young children in the family are excluded. Nevertheless, the ability to understand and work with the cognitive, developmental and psychological processes of all members of a family is crucial for effective and efficient treatment of the whole family unit. That young children represent a unique and valuable contribution to family therapy is an underlying supposition of our work. Our purpose is to demonstrate how young children and their play material contribute to a full understanding of the family and, secondly, show how knowledge of child development and training in child and play therapy are essential to the therapist working with families.

YOUNG CHILDREN'S CONTRIBUTION TO FAMILY THERAPY

The critical functions of the young child as both identified and non-identified patients in family therapy are fully described in a recently published book (Zilbach, 1986). In summary, these functions include:

1. The child as "symptom bearer," providing access to family problems.
2. The child as "tip of the iceberg," displaying difficulties which signal widespread and/or more serious family problems.
3. The child as a therapeutic ally; children are "direct explainers" and can express therapeutic material in uncomplicated words or play, unclouded by adult obfuscation and sophistication.
4. The child as an early detector or barometer of potential problems.
5. The child as crucial participant in the full child-parent-family interactions.

The non-child trained therapist may discover some of these functions by observing overt interactions between the young child and the family, or listening to a verbal child. But if the child is relatively

FAMILY DEVELOPMENT: STAGES OF THE FAMILY LIFE CYCLE

Gestational: "Going Together", Courtship, Engagement

EARLY STAGES: Forming and Nesting

Stage I. Coupling

Family Stage Marker: The family begins at the establishment of a common household by two people which may or may not include marriage.

Family Talk: Individual independence to couple/dyadic interdependence.

Stage II: Becoming Three

Family Stage Marker: The second phase in family life is initiated by the arrival and subsequent inclusion/incorporation of the first child/dependent member.

Family Task: Interdependence to incorporation of dependence.

MIDDLE STAGES: Family Separation Processes

Stage III: Entrances

Family Stage Marker: The third phase is signaled by the exit of the first child/dependent member from the intrafamilial world to the a larger world. This occurs at the point of entrance into school or other extrafamilial environment.

Family Task: Dependence to facilitation of beginning separations-partial independence.

Stage IV: Expansion
  Family Stage Marker: This phase is marked by the entrance of the last child/dependent member of the family into the community.
  Family Task: Support and facilitation of continuing separations-independence.

Stage V: Exits
  Family Stage Marker: This phase starts with the first complete exit of a dependent member from the family. This is achieved by the establishment of an independent household which may include marriage or another form of independent household entity.
  Family Task: Partial separations to first complete independence.

LATE STAGES: Finishing

Stage VI: Becoming Smaller/Extended
  Family Stage Marker: Ultimately the moment comes for the exit of the last child/dependent member from the family
  Family Task: Continuing expansion of independence.

Stage VII: Endings
  Family Stage Markers: The final years start with the death of one spouse/partner and continue up to the death of the other partner.
  Family Task: Facilitation of family mourning. Working through final separations.

Revised from Zilbach, 1968, 1979, 1982, 1986

99

non-verbal, "difficult," or tends to be excluded by the process of family interactions, these functions may remain hidden.

Since the young child is frequently the "symptom bearer," and is often referred for individual psychotherapy, this concept deserves emphasis. Children expressing family pain and difficulties often become the "ticket of admission" to much needed help. In the following example a child therapist's comfort with play material elicited a child's ability to express issues in a poignant and simple way during a family evaluation session.

> A family came to a community clinic because the school principal threatened suspension of the symptom bearer, a twelve-year-old boy. The family was upset by the referral, denying the existence of any difficulties. During the initial family interview, a seven-year-old asymptomatic child quietly sat drawing, apparently absorbed in her play, while the older members of the family continued to maintain their lack of concern. The therapist inquired about the young girl's drawing, thereby treating her contribution as seriously as the parents'. The drawing was a young child's typical representation of a house surrounded by flowers and trees. But tucked away in a window was a tiny figure distinctly saying "help." This simple, clear and important detail provided the entry to an airing of the family's feelings and conflicts surrounding the previously hidden, violent death of an important family member.

It is one thing to acknowledge the contributions of family therapy and more specifically, the contributions that young children can make to family treatment, but it is another to want to work with them and the specific problems they present. At times, sessions truly are harder when they include young children who are frequently fidgety, noisy, distractible, and sometimes obnoxious. Seeing families with one or more young children raises the issues that effective teachers and group leaders must master; mainly, how to keep children under control. At the very least, the therapist must learn some of the techniques that are used by good teachers and group therapists:

As many hands dove into the birthday cake, the therapist disengaged them from the frosting to cut it into equal portions. A food fight threatened, but the therapist controlled it by calmly asking the younger family members to get napkins and distribute plates and cups.

Children inevitably test the therapist's control of the family session. Children often are little "terrors," because they lack mature control over their impulses. At other times, children enjoy the thrill of controlling an adult; and the therapist may fear his/her own impulses as well as fear what the child might do. Limit-setting is crucial and involves the ability to tolerate the child's raw aggression and one's own impulse to retaliate. As Winnicott has taught us, the normal child must strike out at the environment, while the adult must hold and survive (Winnicott, D. W., 1971).

The necessity of recognizing and being tolerant of the ebb and flow of progression and regression as part of normal childhood development is crucial for both child and family work. We have also mentioned the need for therapists to learn ordinary limit-setting and other group therapy skills and interventions. The importance of being familiar with child and adolescent development and with developmentally appropriate avenues of expression and other child experiences is apparent. Yet, with all of these techniques mastered and their advantages recognized, the prospect of including young children in ongoing family sessions may still be uncomfortable. Why? To look for an explanation, we must redirect our attention from what we must learn about children to what we must notice about ourselves as adults. In becoming adults, we banish important elements of childhood. Allying ourselves with children's issues often means dealing with what is repressed in ourselves, and runs counter to the demands of being an adult. Childhood play and fantasies exert a strong regressive pull. One must be able to tap into a child's imagination and to understand the developmental pulls to control and seduce while simultaneously maintaining an empathic alliance with parent care-takers who are likely upset and "troubled" themselves.

As therapists work extensively with children, it is evident how much children struggle to satisfy their own instincts within the family. Therapists with primarily adult training or orientation may see the child as essentially the victim of adult projections. Children are not formed by or just victims of parents. Their powerful instinctual energies are an important family force. Play with children includes playing with the "devil" in them, and the "devil" in oneself; this is uncomfortable and difficult. This primitive nature of children makes us uncomfortable but at the same time is the source of their ability to provide access to the deepest levels of both intrapsychic and family life. Child training teaches the therapist to tap the richness of the child's contribution and to use it in the process of family treatment as well.

Two case examples will illustrate the importance and process of integrating child and family therapy. In both cases the child was symptomatic and referred for psychological evaluation and treatment. The children were seen in weekly individual psychotherapy with ongoing family sessions scheduled approximately once every three to four weeks.

The identified patient in our first example, Beth, a legally blind 14-year-old middle child described herself as: "I'm not the top – I'm not the bottom – I'm the part of the sandwich that's *squeezed* inside and *nobody* can see." Beth's diagnosis of herself is "A zero." She tests in the borderline-average range on a standard I.Q. test with memory difficulties as one outstanding cognitive deficit. Beth's school recommended a psychological evaluation for her. The presenting concerns centered around increased depression, self-destructive behavior, and a question of "bizarre" idiosyncratic behavior. Beth often speaks in numbers and ounces; she has created an intricate rating system which began during early latency – and it became more complicated as she got older. Her numbers all have meanings, and specific people have specific numbers. She has "good" numbers and "bad" numbers and the numbers for her parents change depending on how she's feeling about them, that is, each has a "happy" and "mad" number. About 6 months into her treatment, the therapist discovered that she too had been assigned a number! Beth constantly rates and berates herself – always sitting in judgement of her perceived inadequate performance which is symbolized in her omnipresent rating system. Although Beth provides us with a fascinating case of an individual child with a physical disability, we must resist the temptation of describing the ensuing psychological problems and individual treatment process in more detail and rather focus on the assigned task of demonstrating the importance of integrating individual and family treatment.

As mentioned, Beth has an older and a younger sibling. Because the family lives a great distance from Beth's private school, the parents often come alone for sessions with the identified patient. However, following a number of individual psychotherapy sessions where Beth was recalling some memories around her brother's birth the therapist asked them to bring 5-year-old Andrew for one of the monthly family meetings. Beth entered boarding school at age 8 years and Andrew was born one year later. Beth remembers her mother's pregnancy: "Oh could you help me, my mother would ask. Help her! Help her! If I only knew, I never would have helped her!!" Beth would rail in our individual sessions.

This particular family session began with Beth's usual litany of "all the mistakes I made already today," dramatically showing the three adults where she spilled her toothpaste on her blouse in the morning *and* after lunch! The parents repeated their view that Beth "was not like this before she came to school." They deny remembering her feeling "shy and angry and a behavior problem," although in individual sessions Beth reports memories of being sent to the attic when she was mad and of being toilet trained by her father "who locked me in the bathroom all day until I went on the potty."

Both parents voiced annoyance with Beth's angry defiant behavior when she was home on vacations and wanted to understand where this came from. They began as they had in the past enumerating all of Beth's trouble when she came home. Meanwhile Andrew was disrupting his parents, by throwing Legos and toy cars and running in and out of the office. He ignored his parents' requests to stay in the room and play with the toys provided. Looking at Andrew the therapist began with a discussion of the normal developmental and psychological issues of any 8-year-old daughter who suddenly has a cute little baby brother. At that moment the therapist chose not to elaborate on the expectant reaction of a physically disabled young child with a history of psychologically traumatic hospitalizations and surgery. Beth more poignantly made the point herself. Mother replies: "But she was so excited about the baby, she adored him." Beth blurts out: "Oh, just because he was perfect. Yeah, he didn't weigh just 5 pounds. He wasn't two weeks premature. He could *see*! A perfect stage 8 (the top stage in her system) baby! You didn't need a stage zero daughter anymore since you had a stage 8 baby, so just *go* to school and stay there, we don't need you around anymore!" Beth was angry and crying, and the parents could see and hear, and perhaps sense how abandoned and defective she felt. They could begin to understand her genuine depression and feeling of being replaced by a physically normal, and therefore in the patient's "eyes" perfect and preferred sibling.

Andrew continued to ignore his parents' limits and they began to acknowledge the difficulties they were having with their "perfect" child. For example, he sleeps in his parents' bed almost daily where Beth never came nor was taken into her parents' bed.

With her parents present we talked about Beth's feeling like a zero, "Dr. Gordetsky says I have a giant inferiority complex." It was clarified that although Beth's imaginary number friends appeared before Andrew was born, the "high" numbers, or "angry" numbers developed after he was born.

As the family meeting was ending and the family got up to leave, Beth commented: "You mean I'm so mad at myself for spilling toothpaste because Andrew was born!" thereby making a conscious connection between her intensely felt anger, often displaced onto staff and teachers, and her family dynamics. For not only was a physically normal younger sibling desired and born, but Beth felt and could begin to tell her parents how she perceived him as favored for being "normal" and male. This was not just a distortion on Beth's part, but something the entire family needed to acknowledge and discuss.

This single session exemplifies how Beth's individual psychological issues of low self-esteem, depression and repressed anger is so embedded within larger family issues. The parents, and particularly mother's difficulty in holding this child in esteem despite her physical deficits, is both introjected by the daughter and consciously denied by the mother although frequently unconsciously expressed by the overattentiveness and pride expressed in her other children. This family session, stimulated by the presence of the younger brother, enabled these powerful underground issues to emerge for further family discussion and simultaneously be addressed in continued individual treatment.

The second example, Martin, illustrates the ongoing process of integrating individual child and family treatment and the resulting intrapsychic and family changes that occurred over 6 months of treatment.

Martin is an extremely bright, articulate, 12-year old, who had been taken to his pediatrician on numerous occasions for somatic complaints including headaches, stomachaches and throbbing leg pains without any physical findings. In addition, he began to complain of a sleep disturbance, explaining that the light from his clock kept him awake all night. The actual referral for a psychological evaluation followed a vomiting episode. This latest symptom immediately followed a rare, but explosive, fight between his parents related to his father's drinking too much at a wedding.

Martin's Kinetic Family Drawing shows his parents, Martin, and his 16-year-old sister, Susan riding a roller coaster. This was soon to be viewed as the kind of bumpy course this family experienced on a daily basis, which was both exciting and frightening to Martin. In Martin's initial individual sessions he focused his rage entirely at his sister whom he described as verbally and physically abusive to him; this maltreatment was confirmed by mother as well. At the same time, however, it became clear that there was a sense of admiration for Susan's bold, independent acts toward their parents which indeed represented her maladaptive attempts at separation. Martin also sensed his parents' covert support of his sister's misbehavior when he told a story about a girl who did what she was not supposed to, and her parents were "mad and proud"; the covert support of Susan's acting out "misbehavior" is poignantly illustrated in subsequent family meetings.

After two or three therapy sessions where Martin was seen individually, mother requested a few minutes alone with the therapist. She proceeded to disclose a recent "crisis" and "secret" between

Susan and herself, in which Susan, frightened and tearful, told her mother that she had gone "pretty far" with her boyfriend. Mother requested the names of two additional therapists for herself and her daughter. A family meeting was suggested as an alternative.

First Family Meeting

During the first family meeting, mother and father sat together on the couch. Martin sat in his usual swivel chair next to the therapist, and Susan sat opposite the therapist and between her father and Martin. The mood of the session, as in their household, was dominated by silent, angry treatment from Susan, who chewed gum and rifled through her purse reading pieces of paper she found. Her only verbal comments were nasty remarks made to her brother. The session focussed on the constant fighting between Susan and her father which was perceived as so uncontrollable that the family "could not eat dinner together," and in fact each person ate in a separate room. Mother ate in the downstairs den watching the soap operas she taped all day, Susan ate in her room while she talked on the phone, Martin had his own T.V. to watch, and father ate while reading.

This family as a unit with both children, in early and middle adolescence, were immersed in the family separation process. The individual developmental task of adolescence is to experience themselves as less dependent on their parents and increasingly develop a sense of their own identity, values and goals. The family as a unit must be ready and able to permit, and even gently encourage their adolescents to become invested and have their needs gratified outside the family. Thus this family as a whole was experiencing trouble with the developmental push toward greater separation, and the two children were individually both desirous of and yet uncomfortable with the developmentally appropriate push toward greater individual separation and independence. Martin, the identified patient has developed psychosomatic symptoms that kept him home and close to mother. Susan's provocativeness, a defense against her regressive feelings of dependency and separation anxiety, results in a maladaptive psuedo-separation. The family expresses its developmental arrest by unsuccessfully "ignoring" each other, while in actuality avoiding genuinely working through a gradual, more appropriate, separation.

Individual Session

In the individual session that followed Martin reported having a bad headache the previous evening. When possible precipitants were explored, it was uncovered that Martin lost a cribbage game to his father during dinner — "it was the *second time ever* that I lost!" Martin's conflicts with aggression and competition were similarly apparent in his choice of solitary, non-competitive extra-curricular activities. In early individual sessions Martin sat quietly on a swivel chair and talked with his therapist. When invited to play he often declined or quietly drew pictures. However, within the context of individual psychotherapy sessions Martin slowly allowed hints of his repressed aggression to emerge. First, Martin "dared" to bat around a nerf baseball, gradually hitting it harder and harder against a wall. Later Martin used puppets that pretended to attack his mother during a family therapy session! As Martin felt permission to acknowledge and then explore his ambivalence towards his mother and his internalized conflicts around aggression in general, his symptoms abated. At this juncture mother reported that Martin had slept through the night, but the school was concerned with Susan's behavior and academic performance.

The scenario of a "good child" "bad child" split was present, and this family's need to have a symptomatic child was becoming evident. On an unconscious level, the two children cooperatively took turns providing the "ticket of admission" to treatment for other members of the family and the family as a unit. They knew that unless one of them was a problem, the family would never get help and every family member and the family as a whole would remain developmentally "stuck." In fact, Martin as the initial symptom bearer additionally functioned as the "tip of the iceberg" for widespread individual and family pathology. Despite this family's combativeness and problems, it was as many families, a very caring, loyal family. However, as will become evident, without an actively symptomatic child, the parents would never have sought psychological treatment.

Second Family Meeting

Susan did not come home in time and the family came without her. The session was used to assist the parents in negotiating a reasonable punishment for Susan's disobedience. A significant parental conflict was now unearthed, since father, "the firm one," resisted negotiating *any* punishment because of his conviction that his wife never followed through with any limits on Susan. The mother admitted she felt defeated before she began. Martin, meanwhile, stated that his headaches were gone and he was feeling better. He drew several pictures during this meeting including the first in a series of drawings that will track both Martin's and the family's crumbling defenses. For example, Martin drew pictures of sitting on cloud 9 and rainbows. Over several sessions, the clouds grew grey, then blackened with thunder and rain revealing the anxiety and tension in the family that is about to "pop," as symbolized by the floating and then popping balloons he drew. The other pictures included in the initial family sessions were of a Bloodshot Eye, and his sketch of his mother which he titled, "A Hooker." When the therapist voiced confusion over the picture, which actually looked more like his sister, Martin responded, "My sister in my mother's body." Was the "secret" of Susan's sexual behavior a non-secret?

Third Family Meeting

The parents succeeded in bringing Susan to the next family session where she was given permission to feel angry and remain silent if she wished. Father proudly reported that his wife had grounded Susan the previous Sunday from an afternoon skating outing, and Susan baked cookies for the family instead! Not only was this the first time the family recalled Susan ever initiating such a nurturing task, but both parents seemed incredulous that mother's limits actually worked. Thus the parents, and specifically mother, experienced how setting appropriate limits for Susan were appreciated and furthermore allowed Susan to express affection toward her family, something that had previously been too dangerous, i.e., regressed for an adolescent made anxious by the developmental expectation of separation.

Despite, this family's stated wish "to change" they presented themselves as paralyzed — rationalizing "Susan won't come" or "Susan would refuse." This family had great difficulty negotiating compromises that could meet everyone's developmental and personal needs. For example, after much arguing about New Year's plans they finally acknowledged that it was possible to go out to dinner as a family, and *then* allow Susan to go to a party to be with friends. That this family might want to plan something fun as a family and simultaneously acknowledge the appropriateness of their adolescent daughter wanting to celebrate New Year's Eve with peers, represented a major step toward a more comfortable negotiation of the middle stages of family development and the individual developmental requirements of their two children. Following a celebration as a family Martin, a pre-teen, was happy to spend New Year's Eve with his parents, while Susan preferred and was allowed to be with her friends.

Susan left the family session addressing the therapist for the first time this hour: "I'm not coming back." Mother responds, "Yes, you are, or you'll have to stay in instead." Susan responds, "Well then, I'm *really* going to tell her how I feel, maybe even *swear!*"

Individual Sessions

In the ensuing individual therapy sessions, Martin's intrapsychic conflicts over aggression and separation quickly surfaced. He produced a drawing of a "two-faced rainbow," with clouds and rain replacing his earlier more repressed "cloud 9" drawing, and balloons that were about to "pop" clearly communicated the changes that were observed in Martin, and within the family. For Martin too was about to "pop" as he no longer could easily deny or displace his angry feelings toward his mother. Alone with his therapist, Martin voiced concern about his mother's whereabouts, anxiously wondering what she could and couldn't hear from the waiting room. During another session he observed a wall hanging of an abstract tree with leaves, and suggested that it looked like a boy and a mother who were parts of the same tree, and the boy had a gun and was shooting the mother. This fantasized perception of himself as undifferentiated from his mother "parts of the same tree" and his resultant feelings of anger and anxiety, i.e., do I have to shoot her

in order to separate, confirmed earlier concerns of separation difficulties for Martin who had trouble leaving the therapist's office
each week. The rage, even in fantasy, however, had not been expressed previously. Simultaneously transference issues were explored, as Martin voiced his feeling about the chair he sat in each
week, wondering aloud whether the therapist let other kids sit in it,
too. He described the anger he would feel as he imagined his sister
sitting in it. However, he soon disclosed his recent insight that his
parents had always treated him and his sister differently, with his
sister being pegged the "bad kid" and him as the "good kid." He
began to see Susan's hostility toward him and his attempts at retali-
ation as somewhat misplaced, although the idea that he might be
angry with his mother was still unacceptable to him.

Fourth and Fifth Family Meetings

By the fourth family meeting the seating spontaneously shifted
with Martin giving up his prized "patient" seat to his sister. The
siblings banded together, mischievously throwing the nerf ball back
and fourth, giggling and teasing the therapist. Mother reported that
Martin was sleeping through the night, but he had started talking
back to her!

Mother also reported on things the family did together like going
to a ball game. Significantly mother only purchased 4 tickets rather
than automatically getting an extra so Susan could bring a friend
and dilute the family interactions. The parental couple also went out
"for a whole day alone — just the two of us."

At the end of the session Susan asked how many more sessions
there would be. This was partially interpreted as a question the parents may have wanted to ask and a meeting was set up with the
parents to discuss their treatment. This session clearly illustrated a
shift in the family's intragenerational alliances, a crucial step in
healthy family development. This was apparent as the siblings allied with each other, rather than with one of the parents and fighting
with each other as they had previously done. They also gently
taunted and tested the therapist who was treated via the transfer-

ence, and in reality, as one of "those adults," while the simultaneously emerging strengthened parental alliance was illustrated by mother's casual comment "we went out . . . just the two of us."

Parent Meeting

Both parents perceived many improvements in the family. For example, they were now eating dinner together three times a week. As the therapist raised concerns with Susan's difficulties in school her parents expressed overt support of her school behavior or rather misbehavior. Father stated he had acted similarly in high school and then outgrew it. Mother felt some of the school rules such as no gum chewing were stupid. They were not ready to allow their daughter to give up her maladaptive behavior because of the important role she played in the family, as both the distractor and "voice" of the family's anger and difficulty with control that could only be directed outward onto the school or other external problems or circumstances.

Individual Session

In a following individual session Martin disclosed that he and Susan had a secret talk about him being "the baby in the family," realizing *that's* why he doesn't get punished as much, or for the same things, that Susan does. It appears that once Martin acknowledged this to himself, and admitted this to his sister her anger at him abated and they could ally with each other. Martin repeatedly reminded the therapist not to tell his mother that he knew this. Thus, although their respective roles in the family became very clear to the children, they were consciously willing to continue in them for their parents' sake and for the family as a unit. These children, as most, fear that too much exposure and/or change endangers the continuity of the family; therefore they unconsciously or, as demonstrated here, even consciously behave in ways to maintain the status quo thereby keeping the family together.

Martin strongly denied being interested in the previous week's parent meeting. Instead, in response to some noise from outside the office he fantasized that someone was being thrown against the wall. He was hyper-vigilant concerning his mother's assumed presence or absence in the waiting room; for example, "I think she's gone to the bathroom now."

During this period Martin also reported the following dream: Martin and three friends, 2 boys and 2 girls, one named Sara, were playing together. Sara suddenly turns into ice cubes, then she melts, and he drinks her, and then throws her up.

This dream represents Martin's continued grave conflicts over his wish to introject his sister's aggressive and autonomous parts. However, he becomes so anxious that he immediately needs to exorcise these same attributes. Thus, as a result of Martin's individual intrapsychic shifts, he feels desirous of becoming a more assertive and independent pre-adolescent. However, the family's permission and encouragement in this arena are insufficient to enable him to feel comfortable with his aggression.

Sixth Family Meeting

When the family arrived for their next family session, Susan and her father weren't speaking to each other. As at home, Susan refused to say why she was mad. Finally by whispering to her mother Susan reported being angry at her father for not coming over to her babysitting job when she thought she heard noises in the hall. During this discussion Martin drew a "Freddy is Back" drawing with ominous long, black fingernails, thereby directly expressing what Susan was feeling for her via his drawing. Freddy is the character from the Elm Street horror movies that Susan was watching while she was babysitting. Apparently Susan telephoned father three times to ask him to answer her telephone before she finally was able to make a more direct request for help and protection to which father did not respond. With his scary drawing of the Elm Street intruder, Martin was better able to empathize with his sister's fears and understand her difficulty in asking for help than was father who only saw his daughter as demanding, annoying and self-centered.

Individual Session

Martin arrived at his next individual session clearly agitated, complaining of a headache. He aggressively batted the ball against the office walls exclaiming he did not want to go to dance or religious classes after sessions. He did not tell his mother he didn't want to go, "even headaches won't work, she'll say there's nothing wrong." He told his therapist he couldn't wait to go to summer camp, "to get away from Susan." Thus, Martin, angry and desirous of more autonomy, is still needing to protect his mother and his relationship with her. It becomes clear to both him and his therapist that he feels his need for more control and autonomy will neither be listened to or respected. His role in the family is to be the cooperative child, closely allied with mother, while Susan voices the rebellion and need for separateness which leaves her feeling unprotected and unsafe.

This session was followed by a "terrible week" where Martin spoke back to his mother and was grounded and punished "for the first time ever."

Seventh Family Meeting

Susan and Martin were already fighting over the prized swivel chair as they entered the next family session. Susan read a teen magazine showing her mother pictures and randomly whispering to her father. Martin meanwhile drew "an ugly picture of Susan" and wrote swear words all over it. Martin also gave his sister the finger.

The parents reported that Martin was now consistently sleeping through the night and no longer had headaches; they wondered about termination. Although the therapist agreed that Martin seemed less worried she encouraged the family to continue treatment.

POSTSCRIPT

The parents cancelled the next several family sessions. A family friend was ill and they were spending day and night in the hospital. While the two children were home alone Susan gave herself a superficial cut on her wrist and called her mother, her parents then rushed her to the hospital where psychological treatment was recommended. Thus, now Susan "forced" them to continue treatment, for both herself and the family.

This case illustrates the necessity of integrating individual child and family treatment. Although, both children were clearly symptomatic with serious internalized conflicts over aggression and separation, individual treatment alone would have been insufficient to produce lasting change. For example, although Martin's sleep disturbance and headaches abated quite soon after his individual psychotherapy sessions began, two things emerged immediately to replace these problems. First, Mother began viewing Martin's greater comfort with his aggression as "misbehaving." She reported being alarmed by his "talking back" and refusing to obey her. Second, Susan quickly stepped into the problem child role first by her confiding to her mother she may "have gone too far with her boyfriend," her poor school performance, and when that was not reason enough for the family to continue treatment, she made a suicide gesture. Simultaneous shifts within the family system needed to proceed further before these two youngsters could feel secure enough to relinquish their symptoms. For instance, until the children can sense a more solid parental relationship that could grant genuine permission for direct expression of feelings, difficulties will continue for everyone in the family and "problems" will most likely continue. However, once a stronger parental alliance is established and the parents are committed to seriously listening to every family member's deepest concerns, the children can then afford to relinquish their symptoms and feel more secure about their own individual abilities to proceed developmentally and leave their parents alone together. Thus this case provides us with a striking example of how individual developmental issues such as the ability to feel comfortable with one's own aggression, and ability to feel secure while separating from one's family of origin, is deeply embedded in family developmental issues. Furthermore, unless or until therapeutic interventions address these two different but interrelated developmental systems, change that allows both individual and family development to proceed is not likely. The two case illustrations provide examples of progress in both individual and family development.

REFERENCES

Ackerman, N. (1970). Child participation in family therapy. *Family Process*, 9, 403-410.

Bergel, E., Gass, C., & Zilbach, J. (1968). The use of play materials in conjoint therapy. Proceedings of the IVth International Congress of Group Psychotherapy. *Verlag der Weiner Medizinischen Akademie*, 4-16.

Bloch, D.A. (1976). Including the children in family therapy. In P. Guerin (Ed.), *Family therapy: Theory and practice*. New York: Gardner Press, pp. 168-181.

Chasin, R. (1981). Involving latency and preschool children in family therapy. In A. Gurman (Ed.), *Questions and answers in the practice of family therapy*, Vol. I. New York: Brunner/Mazel, pp. 32-35.

Dowling, E., & Jones, H.V.R. (1978). Small children seen and heard in family therapy. *Journal of Child Psychotherapy* 4 (4), 87-96.

Gordetsky, S., Zilbach, J., & Bennett, M. (1979, April 1). Child therapy—Its contribution to family therapy. Paper presented at the annual meeting of the American Orthopsychiatric Association.

Guttman, H. (1975). The child's participation in conjoint family therapy. *Journal of the American Academy of Child Psychiatry*, 14, 490-499.

Haley, J. (1973). Strategic therapy when a child is presented as a problem. *Journal of the American Academy of Child Psychiatry*, 12, 641-659.

Levant, R.F., & Haffey, N.A. (1981). Integration of child and family therapy. *International Journal of Family Therapy*, 3 (2), 5-10.

Montalvo, B., & Haley, J. (1973). In defense of child therapy. *Family Process*, 12, 227-244.

Tiller, J.W.G. (1978). The specific participation of the child in family therapy. *Journal of the American Academy of Child Psychiatry*, 18, 44-53.

Winnicott, D.W. (1971). *Playing and reality*. New York: Basic Books.

Zilbach, J. (1977, November 5-6). The critical functions of the young child in family therapy. Paper presented at Symposium on the Young Child in Family Therapy. The Psychotherapy Institute and Continuing Education Program, Beth Israel Hospital and Harvard Medical School, Boston, MA.

Zilbach, J. (1982). Young children in family therapy. In A. Gurman (Ed.), *Questions and answers in the practice of family therapy*, Vol. II. New York: Brunner/Mazel, pp. 65-68.

Zilbach, J., Bergel, E., & Gass, C. (1972). The role of the young child in family therapy. In C. Sager, & H.S. Kaplan (Eds.), *Progress in group and family therapy*. New York: Brunner/Mazel, pp. 385-399.

Zilbach, J. (1986) (with Gordetsky, S. and Brown, D.). *Young children in family therapy*. New York: Brunner/Mazel.

TRAINING

Training Therapists to Treat the Young Child in the Family and the Family in the Young Child's Treatment

Connie Moss-Kagel
Robert Abramovitz
Clifford J. Sager

Treating young children in family sessions has been practiced by many therapists since the inception of both child and family therapy without a theoretical base. Now knowledge and practice from psychodynamic theory and family systems, consciously integrated into a unique mode of treating young children and their families, is the content of an eight-week seminar called The Young Child in Family Therapy taught in the Advanced Training Program at the Jewish Board of Family and Children's Services (JBFCS). JBFCS is the agency which resulted when the Jewish Board of Guardians with its

Connie Moss-Kagel, MSW, is Director of the North Brooklyn Office and Instructor, Robert Abramovitz, MD, is Chief Psychiatrist and Codirector, and Clifford J. Sager, MD, is Director of Family Psychiatry and Codirector of Advanced Training Programs, Jewish Board of Family and Children's Services, Inc., New York City.

individual, psychodynamic orientation and the Jewish Family Service with its family systems orientation, merged in 1978 integrating both perspectives in its in-service training and Advanced Training Programs. The purpose of the seminar, The Young Child in Family Therapy, is to expand the participants' assessment and treatment skills with young children and their families by using both family systems and psychodynamic theories and techniques.

This article describes the course, with its integration of current developments in both child and family therapy. We address working on both levels in the treatment of young children: their inner development and the environment (the family) in which they develop, exploring the relationship between the two. Briefly, the seminar covers the prior polarization between family and child therapy, theory which unifies these two poles and practice issues in actually working with young children and their families. However, lest theory be wrenched from its human context, the following paragraph introduces a family we shall refer to throughout the article to illustrate the relationship of the theoretical and the practical with an actual child and her family.

Jane Smith was desperate when she sought therapy for her three-year-old daughter. She was exhausted, confused and guilt-ridden about three-year-old Susan's night terrors and daytime tantrums. Susan was waking screaming in the middle of the night, eyes open but unable to recognize or take comfort from her parents. She cried for up to an hour at a stretch, hitting those trying to comfort her and keeping the household in turmoil. The family pediatrician found no physical basis for this behavior. Jane did not consider including her husband, Mitchell, and her five-month-old son, Max, when she called for an appointment because she viewed the problem as Susan's and an outgrowth of her own inadequacy in parenting. Willingly, she agreed to the suggestion that the whole family attend the initial session. Jane arrived first laden with a diaper bag and two children, Susan and Max. She was harried, but had a sense of humor about the general chaos she and her children created in the waiting room. She was attending to the sunny-faced baby boy while Susan was rooting through the diaper bag, strewing its contents from one end of the large waiting room to the other, demanding gum. When Mitchell walked into this scene twenty minutes late, Susan ran to him with outstretched arms, abandoning her search for gum.

Without being told, selecting the "identified patient" in this scene would be difficult. In fact all of the family members except the infant were in pain, in conflict, struggling with issues in their individual development and in the life cycle of the family. Because of the interconnection of their problems and optimism about the strength in the family members, it was decided that Susan's symptoms could be best treated in family sessions. This choice could not have been as easily made fifteen years earlier because of a polarization between therapists who work with children and those who work with families. We will examine this polarization and a bridging concept.

IS THE WAR ENDING?

The first step in reducing the polarization between child therapy and family therapy is in recognizing that it exists. Guerin (1976) identifying this division in a history of the first twenty-five years of family therapy states that an initial integration of psychodynamic and a systemic perspective in family therapy was lost with the death of Nat Ackerman, one of family therapy's pioneering and revered psychoanalytic proponents. The polarity was reinforced by those working individually with children and became "the undeclared war between child psychiatry and family therapy" (McDermott and Char 1974).

During this period of division there were refinements of psychoanalytic theory and family systems theory. Psychoanalysis expanded from a focus solely on unconscious, id processes to include knowledge about the development of the ego, the object and the self; family systems theory which initially focused on control mechanisms increased its scope to include consideration of those mechanisms which induce change in a system. However, a need for a new way of organizing the complex data from both perspectives exists.

A BASIS FOR DETENTE: THE SHARED METAPHOR

General systems theory is a frame of reference through which the individual and the family can be seen as systems on different levels which do not exclude each other. The accumulated knowledge of individual dynamics does not diminish the power of family systems theory and vice versa. Nichols (1987) points out that "cybernetics and general systems theory provide useful metaphors, helping clinicians become aware of the large movements we rarely appreciate in our own experience." While systems theory is a concept that has generally been associated with family therapy, it is the result of a general shift in scientific perspective emerging over the last few centuries. Ludwig von Bertalanffy (1968) traced the history of science as being one in which we had "atomized" phenomena breaking them down to their smallest parts. He stated that science had "isolated the elements of the observed universe . . . expecting that, by putting them together again, conceptually or experimentally, the whole or system . . . would result and be intelligible. Now we have learned that for understanding, not only knowledge of the elements but their interrelations are required as well . . ." Systems theory is the metaphor science uses to organize the elements and demonstrate their interrelatedness in many fields.

This lens or metaphor for organizing data is used by individual and family therapists to clarify intrapsychic and interpersonal development. Bateson's work is recognized as articulating the development of systems thinking in relation to human behavior (Guerin 1976). Following his lead, family therapy claimed as its own in the field of human relations, exclusive rights to the concept and it was swept into the polarization between family and individual therapists. However, many people associated with individual psychodynamics consciously used the metaphor (Grinker 1956; Menninger 1957; Bowlby 1969, 1973; Peterfreund 1980).

Rene Spitz (1975), without an acknowledgement, applies general systems theory in describing the interchange between mother and infant as "a dialogue of action and response which goes on in the form of a circular process within the dyad as a continuously mutually stimulating feedback circuit." Here he uses the theory of control mechanisms founded on the concepts of information and feedback in systems showing self regulation and the capacity for change, to describe physical and interpersonal development which results from interchanges between mother and infant. Only using this metaphor could he convey the complexity of the interaction and the subsequent intrapsychic and interpersonal patterns in the dyad. Spitz and also Stern (1977) demonstrate the bridging power of systems thinking in their formulations. Though they confined their remarks to the mother-infant unit or the dyad in the above described works, systemic thinking can be applied to all ages and all intimate relations *to explain both intrapsychic development and family systems or relations*, using the same metaphor.

Family therapists use the same language and concepts as Stern and Spitz with all members in the family. In family systems thinking every behavior is a communication which stimulates a feedback of another behavior communication (Watzlowick et al. 1967). Mara Selvini Palozzoli et al. (1978) apply the term "circularity" to the family. They see the family as a "self regulating system which controls itself according to rules formed over a period of time through a process of trial and error . . . which comes to exist through a series of transactions and corrective feedback." All of these theorists use systems language to describe not only the people but the interrelations between people as vital points of observation.

We are not denying differences but rather pointing out the larger lens used by all of these theorists which provides us with a unifying, organizing principle. Systems theory is a frame of reference through which the individual and the family can be seen as systems on different levels not concepts which oppose each other. Nichols (1987) points out that "family therapy has moved too far from the individual, resulting in a wave of esoteric theorizing and proliferation of mechanistic, highly technical interventions." The same could be said for individual formulations that refuse to look at the developments of the last thirty years in understanding families. There is a need to move back toward a center point without losing the contributions of family therapy or losing the advances in psychoanalysis.

THE LOCUS OF THE PROBLEM:
THE EXTENDED METAPHOR

One of the traditional areas of conflict between individual therapists and family therapists is the question of where the problem resides: in the individual or in the family? No one disputes that troubled families produce troubled individuals and vice versa. Not until recently, however, has there been a comprehensive approach that attempts to clarify in an organized way the relationship between the two. A problem or a symptom will exist in the individual, in the family and in the relationship between them.

Individual therapists look primarily at the child's development and psychic structure while family therapists primarily examine the interactions in the family. In an excellent article describing the treatment of a child Anna Ornstein (1976) focuses on "developing empathy" in a parent, for a child's anxiety but does not reflect an understanding of how the child's symptom functioned in the relation to the mother's psyche or to a remarried family. On the other hand, Donald Bloch (1976) in an article on child focused family therapy recognizes the developmental issues of the child and then proceeds with an example which does not reflect the developmental complications implicit in a mother sitting on her jealous son. Addressing the problem or the symptom on one or the other level alone may facilitate some change fostering the development of one family member, but leaving the others untouched or changing the family at the expense of individual development. Understanding the function of a symptom on all levels opens the options for effective intervention.

Terms are already in use that demonstrate the relationship between the intrapsychic and the family system. Spitz (1975) uses the phrase "derailment of the dialogue" and Stern (1977) uses the phrase "missteps in the dance" to describe patterns of communication which thwart individual development and interpersonal relations in the dyad. Both of these phrases indicate that the locus of the problem is not an either-or proposition: it resides in the individuals and in their interaction.

Carlos Sluzki (1981) describes a symptom tracking method which can be used to show in action the "derailment of the dialogue" or the "missteps in the dance" between the individual and the family members. He says, "the symptom proper is considered one link of a mutual-causal sequence without end. Special attention is placed on which behaviors of the symptom-carrier and/or of the family members are generated and suppressed by the symptoms." In treating the family or individual we use the symptom and family members' reaction to it as the beginning point of discussion and as the sign of movement in the ongoing treatment. A symptom is frequently what the individual or family presents as the problem with the content of sessions focusing on it. But it is also much more; it is an active expression of the attempt to achieve a balance between forces intrapsychically and systemically. To draw on psychoanalytic theory, it is overdetermined or has multiple functions. Intrapsychically, a symptom is a failed attempt to balance functions of the personality—the ego, the id, and the superego. In a family, a symptom (usually the behavior or feelings of one family member and conflict in the family) is a failed attempt to maintain a balance among members or units in the family. In both cases it is an attempt to be all things and meet all needs for people: its ultimate role is to attempt to provide an intrapsychic and interpersonal harmonious balance. But the symptom is not the problem. *A symptom is a failed attempt to solve a problem.* The problems to be remedied by putting the "dialogue on track" or eliminating the "missteps in the dance" are restated in the following:

1. pain in individuals
2. conflict in the family
3. conflict with the community
4. impediments to the individual's movement through the stages of development (the individual's life cycle phases)
5. impediments to the family's movement through the family life cycle or family development.

The question then arises, if symptoms function on both levels and on the interaction between the levels, how does a therapist decide on which level to intervene? The late Dr. Stanley Lesser, formerly chief psychiatrist at JBFCS, taught that the level of therapeutic focus is determined by the point of greatest leverage for change, for which basic knowledge of each level is a prerequisite.

WHAT KNOWLEDGE IS NECESSARY TO WORK WITH CHILDREN IN FAMILY THERAPY OR FAMILIES IN CHILD THERAPY?

Advanced trainees wishing to treat children and their families need the following initial knowledge of both individual and family development and behavior prior to attempting an integration.

1. individual life cycle, particularly child development
2. the family life cycle
3. family systems
4. the relationship of individual symptoms to the family and vice versa
5. an understanding of one's self and family of origin

With ninety years of writing about the nature of the psyche and thirty-five years of writing about the family from which to draw, the beginning therapist can feel overwhelmed about mastering this body of knowledge. We would have no therapists if immediate mastery were a requirement. Becoming a therapist is a lifelong, dynamic process of development. The following discussion of each point serves as a guide in the process of becoming a therapist who treats young children and their families.

1. Individual Life Cycle

We absorb the perspectives on individual development from our own upbringing and people close to us. People contemplating becoming therapists consciously consider their own development and that of others. Our personal experience is probably the primary basis for our assumptions about development. Personal therapy enables the therapist to fully articulate and examine with another his own assumptions. Education enables us to evaluate our own assumptions by comparing them with those of people recognized as astute observers and clear thinkers. The untreated therapist who ignores the contributions on development puts the client at the mercy of his/her implicit, unexamined theory of development.

Some of these clear thinkers and astute observers are worth highlighting here. Sigmund Freud first outlined the stages of the drives. Heinz Hartman working from Freud began to delineate the importance of the ego. Greenberg and Mitchell (1983) describe the many significant contributors to object relations theory. Heinz Kohut elaborates theories of the development of the self. Anna Freud (1981), in addition to her contributions on the ego, gave us a way of organizing and applying this diverse information in her concept of lines of development. This concept allows one to trace normal development along a number of lines defined by her father and other contributors establishing a base line by which to evaluate development.

Infant researchers are currently augmenting and refining our understanding of development. It is not possible to do justice to all the contributions to developmental theory here. Our goal is to point out an initial approach using developmental lines to organize a new therapist's thinking about individual human psychological development. It is also important to highlight specific lines of development that are essential to working with children in individual or family treatment. Without going into a full discussion of cognitive development, the exploration of how children communicate, particularly in play, is a specific knowledge that is basic to working with them.

Katan (1961) describes the following characteristics of children's verbalization

A. Verbalization of perception of the outer world precedes verbalization of feelings.
B. Verbalization leads to an increase of the controlling function of the ego over affects and drives.
C. Verbalization enables the ego to distinguish between wishes and fantasy on one hand, and reality on the other. In short, verbalization leads to integration which in turn results in reality testing and thus helps to establish the secondary process.

More age appropriate verbalization in sync with emotional development is both a goal of development and therapy. The lack of language skill should not, however, eliminate the inclusion of young children in therapy either individually or in family sessions. To do so would equate language singularly with communication and eliminate the context in which language is developed, modified, expanded and meaning agreed upon. Verbalization is preceded by nonverbal means of communication but is never entirely substituted for it at any stage of development. Play is an important life-long, nonverbal, means of communication.

Harter (1983) describes play as the therapeutic analogue of free association with adults. Winnicott (1971) states that "playing can be a form of communication in psychotherapy." It may be the primary way that children communicate their deepest feelings in any circumstance. Peller (1954) applied these observations to developmental theory by delineating for each age and stage common concerns that children partialize to master. The central theme of all play in her scheme is object relations at its various stages; play is a way of working through previously unmastered issues in relation to the self and the object based on the stage of development. Peller presents this information in a way that the beginning therapist can use to anticipate the concerns and modes of communicating of children at any stage. Play has an important function in families in maintaining health and promoting growth. Playing with children in sessions enhances family playfulness in general through which many issues in families can be negotiated. Griff (1983) created a model of family play therapy which serves as an adjunct to the ongoing treatment in which new adult learning theories are applied. This brief review of individual development provides an outline of knowledge necessary for assessment, intervention and monitoring individual development.

2. Family Life Cycle

The family life cycle is the predictable, observable stages which families go though over time: it is comparable to the normal individual phases of development through which all individuals pass on the way to maturity. The usual stages and tasks described by the family life cycle are coupling, the first child, the expanded family, individualization of family members, separation of younger members, the shrinking family and finally the death of one and then both partners. A knowledge of the family life cycle provides the beginning therapist a tool to assess the family and monitor its progress in treatment in the same way that knowing individual development serves for the individual. It provides a base line to determine the stage of the family and normative issues during that stage. A number of theorists have delineated the stages of family development (Zilbach 1986; Carter and McGoldrick 1980; Haley 1973; Rhodes 1977). Sager et al. (1981, 1983) did the same for the remarried or stepfamily system.

Like our understanding of individual development, our assumptions about the family life cycle start early. We have attitudes about a variety of life cycle issues. A knowledge of others' theories enables us to put our own experience and assumptions in the context of a larger view, keeping the universal and abandoning that which is idiosyncratic.

The value of understanding the family life cycle can be demonstrated in two events in the Smith family. First, Jane's establishing her own family at age forty shortly after the death of her own parents is prompted by an attempt to replace them rather than mourn their loss and is not just a reflection of a change in life cycle trends toward having families later in life: it is a faulty personal adjustment with potential sequelae. The birth of a second child is also a normative life cycle issue that evoked extreme stress in this family. The mother's depression emerged, the father's conflicted role as primary provider became accentuated with his wife not working and daughter responded with normal feelings of rivalry and extreme demands for attention. The "derailment" of life cycle responses could be gauged because there is a knowledge of the normative life cycle.

3. Family Systems

Family systems theory was highly controversial and misunderstood initially. The controversy stemmed in part from family systems' departure from the model of psychotherapy current at the time by conceptualizing and treating the individual's symptoms in the context of the family, and in the case of some theorists, ignoring individual dynamics altogether. Misunderstanding also resulted from the use of language that previously had not been associated with human behavior. Terms like "feedback," "input," and "output" had the ring of the physical sciences. Like the concepts of the "id" the "ego" and the "superego," the language of family systems is confusing if reified rather than used as a metaphor which allows discussion of complex interrelationships within the family. Controversy was also stimulated by family therapists themselves as an outgrowth of "boundary functions" to use a systems term or establishing their identity as those of an analytic bent might say. We have arrived at a time when the legitimacy of family systems has been established so that this struggle can be relinquished. Family systems contribution can be combined with those of psychodynamic theory to advance our understanding and treatment of people.

The following are ideas basic to family systems thinking. A family is more than the sum of the individuals who make it up and has interactions which are unique, specific and repetitive that have evolved over time. The exchanges in a family become internalized in its members insuring that they become patterns. If one family member changes, there are corresponding changes in other family members. Finally, if a family member is designated as symptomatic, the symptom and even the designation of being symptomatic are meaningful and functional in the exchanges in the family.

When sitting in the room with a family, knowing that all interchanges are meaningful prevents us from dismissing ones that elucidate the family rules and interaction.

> Three-and-a-half-year-old Susan who randomly said "poop, poop, poop" throughout the Smith's mid-afternoon sessions was dismissed as being ill-mannered and attempting to annoy her parents, Jane and Mitch. While her behavior had meaning on a developmental level (she regressed back to diapers after the birth of her brother) and a communications level (it interrupted the parents' discussion) it was also reflective of the family difficulty and current reality. At one point she asked to be taken to the bathroom which the therapist did at the request of her weary parents. Susan proceeded into the booth and had a bowel movement. Afterward the therapist asked her if she

was saying "poop because she had to go poop." She assented. When the parents were told of this conversation, the mother said that Susan regularly had a bowel movement at this time of day but she had not recognized the signal of her need.

This incident reflects the overwhelmed parents' difficulty with their daughter's needs. Susan did not say "poop" in the session after she returned. Because of parental stress on other levels and their subsequent lack of energy, they labeled and responded to three-year-old Susan's signal of a basic need as though it were misbehavior on which the parents then discharged their own frustrations. Should this derailment of the dialogue persist, Susan will be confused about her bodily products, perceptions and interactions. She will not develop reliable ways of signaling those she depends on to meet her needs and therefore interactions will become distorted.

4. The Relation of the Individual Symptoms to the Family and the Family Symptoms to the Individual

The relationship of symptoms between each level is relatively unexplored in the literature. Herschkowitz and Kahn (1980) proposed a model integrating psychoanalytic structural theory and family systems in which the degree of psychic structuralization in each family member mirrors the level of autonomous functioning of the family. Brighton-Cleghorn (1987) integrates self psychology and family systems theory to demonstrate that in a family which uses a child as a "self object" or a way of meeting its own needs, this disorder will be reflected as a self disorder in the internal world of the child.

An examination of the issue of resistance further clarifies the relationship between the intrapsychic and the interpersonal levels. Strean (1985) describes how Freud and Breuer a hundred years earlier looked at resistance as an intrapsychic process in which there is an avoidance of danger by the patients separating unbearable ideas from the rest of their ideational life and from their free associations as if these ideas were not part of themselves. Lerner and Lerner (1983) looking at resistance from a systemic approach agree that it reflects intrapsychic function and transference but in addition they think that there may be real consequences in a client's family if he/she relinquishes a symptom. A familiar example of these consequences is that of codependency in an alcoholic's family. Frequently when an alcoholic abstains from drinking the intrapsychic and interpersonal problems of other family members emerge. In other words a resistance to change may have both important intrapsychic and familial bases. Psychoanalysts view symptoms as efficient, addressing a number of intrapsychic components. This efficiency seems to extend to the external world also: a symptom may preserve an intrapsychic balance and balance in a family.

5. An Understanding of One's Self and Family of Origin

This understanding is, as mentioned earlier, a life long endeavor. References to this are interspersed in other sections throughout this chapter. (Also see Bennett & Zilbach, pp. 145-157 and Kramer, pp. 173-185.)

FROM THEORY TO PRACTICE IN TREATING YOUNG CHILDREN IN FAMILY SESSIONS

From theory we now move into actual treatment with several areas of special consideration:

1. the room and materials
2. bridging different levels of communication
3. removing the child from the marital conflict
4. parental empathy and limit setting
5. who should be in the room
6. sitting with the family
7. the primary intervention.

1. Room and Materials

The room should be large enough, comfortable and childproof. The therapist should include materials and toys that are age appropriate but will not in themselves become the focus. For all ages, toys that are safe, stimulate interaction or enhance communication of the child's feelings are desirable.

For children under three one might have a toy they can push around the room, a cuddly toy, toys that require dexterity (rings of graduated size and a stick), a baby doll and a car. Noisy toys have an obvious disadvantage in family therapy sessions particularly if the session is being recorded. Toys or material that requires cleanup have both advantages and disadvantages. For children under three there are significant developmental and interpersonal issues related to being clean or dirty which can be addressed in the session when water, Play-Doh or other materials are used (see Peller [1954] for a review of developmental issues).

Use and desirability of these materials needs to be decided on a case by case basis. For example, in addition to fostering the child's development, cleaning up the toys at the end of the session is one of the integral parts of using them in these sessions. It allows "in vivo" a demonstration of the family's capacity to carry out tasks. If this is a very conflicted area, using messy materials may elicit struggles that the new tenuous therapeutic alliance cannot contain. Finally, when the practitioner has therapy sessions back to back, even with the best family cleanup, there may not be adequate time to prepare the room for another session. There may be alternate ways to address the same issues in the family if "messy play" is not feasible.

For the three- to six-year-old child, many of the same materials are used. However at this age they are more capable of sustained play creating their own story. They can use doll houses, garages with cars, dress-up material and Play-Doh. Their play frequently reflects on or elaborates their feelings about the adult conversation as well as their own preoccupation. They hear what is happening in the session. While children at this age may not be able to organize and express their thoughts like adults do, they are able to talk about some feelings and give their version of an event. The elaboration of feelings and thoughts is primarily expressed in nonverbal means but verbalization can be elicited and meaning confirmed.

The materials for seven- to eleven-year olds overlap with those used by the younger children depending on the child. Most articles describing therapy with children in family therapy are written about this age. Different from younger children who may not have the cognitive ability to fully articulate feelings and thoughts verbally but who are uninhibited, this age child may have newly formed defenses which are unsettled by open communication. Whatever play materials are used, they should respect his/her tenuously developing ability at mastery and the need to maintain recently developed defenses. Zilbach's (1972, 1986) use of drawings, Guttman's (1975) use of spontaneous behavior in sessions, and Villeneuve's (1979) use of sculpting, and psychodrama are all play techniques that require few toys and very basic materials.

The use of toys and materials functions in two ways. First, they should provide the material to enhance the ability of all family members to communicate. Second, through the use of toys a playfulness can be established in the session creating a pleasant, easy atmosphere for family members to resolve issues and to serve as a model for an easier, more joyful environment for all members.

2. Bridging Levels of Communication

The ways that therapists have tried to bridge the difference in communication levels is as varied as the people doing it. In addition to language, people communicate in a variety of ways. Their tone of voice, posture, where they sit in relation to others, motoric discharge, and their affect all communicate. The four primary ways that have been used by those working with young children in family therapy are:

A. Interpreting the spontaneous behavior of children which reflects their feelings and thoughts in reaction to what is said or done in the session. For example, after stopping Susan from pinching Max the therapist says "You're angry with Mommy and Max because Mommy is feeding him and not playing with you."

B. Using organized activities which allow all members to participate including young children. Sculpting, psychodrama and audiovisual techniques are some of the activities used in this way.

C. Using drawing in the session enabling children a means of responding to the conversation in the session and as a tool which can be used to convey their reactions and heighten

parents' awareness of their children's feelings. This is an activity that seems to work best with latency age kids.

D. Listening and responding in an age appropriate way to the
child's verbal communications, recognize his/her presence
and communicate rapport and understanding: In the Smith
family, Susan was remarkably able to describe her version of
feelings and events leading to a tantrum which gave the parents insight into her reactions and options for responding to
them. These activities can be between parent and child or
therapist and child or between children.

A therapist who is comfortable with and understands children's
communication can use this knowledge. A simple game of peeka-
boo with an infant can establish contact with that child, serve as an
aid in assessing the child's development, elicit the parents' comfort
in interacting with their child, nurture the family by proxy, and
change the tone of a family session from a fearful search for a problem to a relaxed joining in the search for solutions. Playfulness in
itself is a goal which such communication can encourage. These
techniques are not simply geared to elicit information. They should
also serve to provide the parents with tools for relaxed interchanges
and problem solving outside of therapy. Age appropriate verbal participation of all family members is a goal in working with children.
It is not, however, a prerequisite for being included in therapy sessions.

3. Removing the Child from Roles in Marital Conflict

One contribution of family therapy is the idea of removing the
identified client from the role of symptom bearer for the family.
Haley (1973) addressing the issue of the symptomatic child, says
that one of the parents is overinvolved and the other is more periph-
eral. While other family therapists may take issue with this specific
formulation, there is general agreement that marital dysfunction interferes with parenting. One of the ways of attempting to remove
the child from that position is to reframe or positively connote the
child's behavior to alter the family's thinking and reactions about
him/her. While frequently effective when done with a clear understanding of the symptom's function in the system, this intervention

must not be used in a way that denies and ignores a child's developmental issues.

There are several other ways to address this issue in the family. One is through the relationship: the therapist joins the family system and begins to be used in the way that the family, particularly the conflicted marital couple, incorporates any third person. This joining of the system usually provides relief and a challenge to the symptomatic child in itself. When this happens, the child must be supported in handling age and stage needs appropriately which were previously met by being triangulated. They can get this support in an altered relation with parents or/and with a therapist, siblings, friends or in school. They can continue to be seen in family sessions in order to work through their new role in the family and participate in their parents' new attempts to resolve old problems without triangulating the child. The therapist then provides the couple with the missing functions while helping them become aware of what these needs are and developing mechanisms to meet them in a way that does not hamper individual family members' development or the movement of the family through its life cycle.

For example:

> Jane Smith's unresolved mourning for her parents is aggravated by Mitch's withdrawal to which she reacts with anger, fear of abandonment and increased dependency. When she is needy she spends a great deal of time with three-year-old Susan, indulging her to meet her own dependency needs. When Mitch again becomes available to her, Jane turns to him without weaning Susan from the level of attention her own dependency stimulated. Susan reacts with increased demands. Jane protecting Mitch from her anger by displacing it on to Susan, responds angrily to her demands. Susan responds to her mother's anger with tantrums which Jane cannot control requiring Mitch to intervene. Mitch is also uncomfortable in directly expressing his frustrations at Jane's demands for intimacy and support which he experiences as overwhelming. He too discharges his anger at his daughter rather than his wife using harsh methods in bringing Susan under control. His harshness makes Jane angrier with him and more guilt-ridden about dis-

placing it on Susan. She then undermines Mitch's discipline which permits the child to become further out of control. Susan (in addition to accommodating her parents' need to rationalize their harshness) is at a stage where she too desires a closer relationship with her father and will continue to have tantrums to maintain an attachment to him since his withdrawal from the family provides her with no modified avenue for a relationship with him.

Since this family came to therapy seeking help with their child's tantrums, to start with any other issue would be experienced as threatening and unempathic. If both parents were able to deal with a direct expression of underlying problems in the marriage and the affects engendered in response to those problems they would not be seeking therapy. Thus the therapist must start with the tantrums. To intervene to change the tantrums alone however, unless that intervention takes into account the multiple levels on which that problem exists, is not helpful. It may reinforce the child's role as scapegoat and result in a symptom substitution in which the child accommodates the parents' needs to continue to displace their anger and act out their difficulty with intimacy without addressing their relationship. The tantrums had to be addressed within the child, and in the family system. Understanding the relationship of her tantrums to the marital relationship, the mother's overinvolvement and father's withdrawal, father's paucity of constructive interaction with his daughter and the parents' lack of techniques to change undesirable behavior, aided in taking steps that reduced the tantrums significantly and eliminated the night terrors.

4. Facilitating Parental Empathy and Limit Setting

Empathy and limit setting are not just child rearing techniques: they are ways of relating that all family members need to learn. When parents bring children to treatment they are frequently seeking limit setting techniques. Therapists are frequently the ones who define lack of parental empathy as a problem. The topic of empathy and limit setting have been combined because neither should spring from love or anger although to ignore the involvement of these affects would not be realistic: they should arise as a response to developmental needs and reality. When harshness or unresponsiveness is a problem in the family, it exists on all levels. If father is rough with the children and mother does not mediate his harshness and sisters and brothers tell on each other, everyone is in need of limits and empathy as well as needing to control themselves and be empathic.

The therapist's communication to family members will be the basic model of empathy family members will absorb as an alternative to their family patterns. Sitting in a room and responding supportively and evenly to each member of a family in which people are in pain, angry with each other and feel defeated in their own attempts to correct these problems, provides the family with nurturance and a model to emulate. It is hard to listen to a mother who is angrily telling a four-year old that the dog he accidentally let out of the house is probably dead and the mother can see that the son doesn't care that the pet that mother loved so much is gone. It is easy to become angry with the mother and want to rescue the child. The difficulty is compounded when father condones mother's harshness by omission or commission. The empathic model is to respond to each person's feelings about the incident. The responsibility for controlling impulses, their own and their children's resides with the parents which is where the focus in the session may be. However, the foundation for that work is in understanding the meaningfulness of a symptom for all family members individually and in relation to each other.

Oldens (1961) thinks that a child's pull to regression on the mature ego of the parent puts stress that only a flexible ego can withstand. She points out that conscious or unconscious aggression and anxiety, narcissistic disappointment or withdrawal all complicate parents' empathy with a child. Her recommendation for personal analysis is not immediate or practical for parents who are struggling with tantrums now. There are several ways to address this differently with parents. If the parents are motivated and insightful, parent guidance can be helpful. Samlin's (1987) book on positive discipline is helpful. She has a number of alternatives to the use of punishment. Her discussion of age appropriate needs of a child and possible responses to those needs aids parents in avoiding damaging conflict.

Usually by the time a family seeks therapy, patterns are already entrenched and maladaptive. The maladaptive patterns are repeated because they are meaningful to all members and serve a function in the family system. Nichols (1987) suggests that we can teach empathy using Murray Bowen's technique of interviewing an individual in a family session, keeping our responses genuine but short so that other family members are not blocked by a preoccupation that their needs will not be met. Stierlin et al. (1980) view Boszormenyi-Nagy's concept of "multidirectional partiality" as an extension of the idea of empathy. Equal attention in a session is not always possible, but as Stierlin et al. say, "the therapist must convey to each [family member] the feeling that she or he is a worthwhile person, somebody who counts and whose position the therapist is trying to understand and respect."

5. Who Should Be in the Session?

At assessment all family members should be seen together because every member influences and is influenced by the family. The young child, even if an infant, must be present with the family. We learn from who holds, relates to, cares for, indulges or ignores the young child. The child need not be the identified patient. His presence provides us with much useful information about him and his family. Seeing all family members initially is also important in order to determine whether the family's designation of one person as the identified patient is part of a pattern of scapegoating and hence resistance which the therapist does not want to reinforce. Individual assessment sessions afterward are also necessary. The ultimate choice of treatment modality is based on a knowledge of the individuals' and family members' interaction.

A young child is included in family therapy sessions when her/his exclusion would reinforce a denial of his role in the family or the family's role in the child's problems and when the parents and the child or children have the capacity to alter patterns of interactions or put the dialogue back on track. Family therapy with small children can be the primary mode of treatment or it can be ancillary to the individual treatment of any family member or marital treatment. Used as an adjunct to the individual therapy of a child, it can address environmental issues in which the parents' response to the child is crucial.

> In the individual treatment of a 10-year-old boy whose father had died suddenly of cancer two years before, his 53-year-old mother was seen in six conjoint sessions to help him tell her that her drinking in the evening raised the fear in him that he would lose both parents. Despite this mother's resistance to therapy for herself to mourn the loss of her husband, she was able to hear her son's underlying concern and respond reassuringly by reducing her drinking.

In marital therapy in which the child becomes triangulated, or locked into an inappropriate role in the parents' relationship, the child needs to be seen to assess the situation. If the child is functioning and on track developmentally, the therapist may want to see him/her briefly to help all members change the way they interact but then see the parents for marital therapy.

There are certain conditions under which young children should not be seen in family sessions. If a child is in individual treatment and the trust of the child in the therapist will be threatened by conjoint sessions, family sessions with the same therapist are not recommended. This possibility is more likely with adolescents than younger children. If there are separate therapists, consultation with the other therapist clarifies roles. Contraindications for inclusion of a child may be due to the other therapist's theoretical position, or view of your role as competitive. Where multiple modalities are indicated, the question of whether it is appropriate for the therapist to conduct the individual and family therapy or to involve a second therapist is one that needs to be addressed on a case by case basis.

The primary reason for not seeing a child in the family is scapegoating. When the family's scapegoating of a child outstrips their capacity to change the scapegoating behavior to the detriment of the child, then individual treatment is recommended. In this instance different approaches to the family's behavior must be used. While it is true that the child experiences this behavior twenty-three hours a day when not in session, and may himself contribute to the pattern, therapy needs to be a haven where hope resides. The child and the family members may need to be seen individually or in marital therapy for a period of time. Non-destructive family sessions may be an outcome of individual therapy in some cases.

6. Sitting in the Session with Young Children and Their Families

Parents are not the only ones whose ego must be flexible enough to tolerate the regressive pulls of a young child. In addition to sitting in an unknown family and trying to figure out the rules that govern what looks like random interaction to the new therapist, the requirement is to interact on many different levels. If there is a circumstance in which we will revert to old comfortable patterns of coping, this is it. In fact, the therapist who does so, and is aware of his reversion so he can change it in response to the family he/she is treating, finds the beginning stages of this type of therapy easiest. Until a therapist begins to develop his or her tools in the sessions, he needs to rely on his own interpersonal skills using supervision to begin to evaluate which ones are helpful and which ones are not.

7. The Primary Intervention

Families have a tendency to bring in the same issue or variations on an issue repeatedly in their description of the problem. This tendency to repeat is monitored and used to aid the family. The therapist starts where the family is, at the point of the presenting problem. Each person in the family tells his version of the story or the presenting problem. Starting in this way begins to shift the family from seeing one member as problematic to seeing the relationship of each member's problems, feelings and behavior to that of each other and the family as a whole. Family members' versions of the story and their interaction in the session are the therapeutic focus.

Young children hear and have responses to the issues in the family and in the session but some may not be able to make a coherent verbal response. It is at this point that the therapist begins to observe and interpret the varying levels of communication in the family sessions in order to stimulate the development of new observational skills in the family members. All people use nonverbal means of communication. Because young children are less able to communicate verbally they are more dependent on nonverbal means of communicating.

The repetition of the story and the pattern of interaction over many sessions is helpful to the bewildered therapist who is flooded with data in sessions giving him/her many opportunities to understand and intervene and change interventions when they don't work or produce undesirable outcomes. The repeated pattern also gives a baseline against which to measure gains in therapy. There are some "aha" experiences in this therapy but the majority of change is in incremental shifts in a current family's patterns which allow individual and family development to proceed. The recurrent patterns of interaction that emerge in these sessions illustrate the gradual shifts in the family:

> In the first session with the Smith family the three-year old initially used the session to relax on her father's lap while her parents described her tantrums and night terrors which had intensified since her brother's birth. When her mother began to breast feed her five-month-old brother, she left her father's lap and began to move around the room never moving too far from her parents. The farthest she went was to the male and female anatomically correct dolls across the room. She picked up the male doll, taking it back to her mother. After examining its genitals, she then asked her mother to take her to the bathroom (where presumedly she examined her own genitals). When she returned, Susan stayed near her mother and brother poking and pinching him until the mother handed him to the father. The therapist then asked her if she knew how boys were different from girls. Susan replied that boys have a penis. She then tried to physically block the therapist from talking to her mother. Her parents began to describe her as unmanageable at which point she made a face that looked like she was going to be unmanageable but in fact was open to benign influence.

This brief description of interactions in the first session with this family highlights those that repeated in the following sessions. The parents were concerned about controlling her behavior without really understanding it. They discharged their anger at her rather than addressed her concerns. They were locked in this pattern for reasons described previously. Susan was announcing her concerns by her repetitive behavior some variation of which emerged in every subsequent session. She wanted closeness with her father. She was angry about sharing her mother. She regarded her brother as an interloper. She was also concerned about her body and the difference between her body and that of her brother. She wanted to know where babies come from. These issues and the patterns in which they emerged in sessions are repeated in every session. The goal is to acknowledge each individual's communication and the family's characteristic pattern of responding in order to increase awareness and provide a model and experience that is affectively and behaviorally different from previous patterns. In the Smith family, the three-year old's communications about her concerns were repeatedly responded to as "misbehavior." This pattern gave way to an altered response in the course of therapy.

The family structure often affects the way that the problems unfold in therapy. In a two-parent family, it is not unusual for the therapist to be triangulated into the parents' conflict in a similar way to the triangulation of the symptomatic child, a move that indicates a level of engagement as well as a resistance to acknowledging the conflict between the marital couple and the impact it has on the children. In single-parent families, it is likely that the parent will initially use the therapist to provide an aspect of parenting that is missing in the family. Single mothers frequently want the therapist to be limit setting with their children and single fathers want the therapist to be nurturing to their child. These expectations are in the service of actually having the need met rather than acknowledging the deficit in the family and doing the necessary problem solving about an ongoing way to meet those needs—the ultimate task in therapy. While initially accepting these roles, it is essential that the therapist move the family toward acknowledging the nature of the missing functions in the family so that the family can ultimately become independent of the therapy. Sager et al. (1981, 1983) describe the way that the treatment of the remarried family unfolds towards this goal.

Infants should be included in sessions also. Their exclusion limits understanding of them and their role in the family. Problems inherent in excluding an infant from the assessment became particularly apparent in a family of four sons in which the father was diagnosed as having terminal cancer. Their mother said she regretted having her last child, a two-year-old boy, who was not discussed in the assessment nor included in the sessions. His exclusion is indicative of some acting out of the mother, the impact of which on the infant's development and the family needed to be assessed.

In the instance of our Smith family, the periodic inclusion of the infant soon was essential to assess his needs and understand the family. As he moved closer to age two and his sister's problems subsided, the Smiths became concerned about his behavior. His presence in the session also stimulated his sister's enactment of her specific response to him, and gave a live demonstration of the strengths of the parents in their sensitive, responsive parenting in the first year of life in addition to the developmental points at which they might have difficulty. Finally, his periodic presence gave a baseline by which to measure the family's progress in working through the issues stimulated by his birth.

IN CONCLUSION

Had the Smith family seen a therapist ten years ago, Susan's tantrums and night terrors would have been treated from only one of the poles in the field at the time. If the family had seen a child therapist, the symptoms indicating intrapsychic conflict would have been treated leaving the family configuration which reinforced them untreated, and other family members in pain, laying the groundwork for symptom substitution in Susan or other family members. If a family therapist was the consultant, the likelihood is that the underlying marital conflicts and consequent disturbance in parenting would be addressed without treating the intrapsychic and developmental disturbance in the child or other family members.

General systems theory provides a metaphor which does not require a choice between perspectives. Rather, contributions from individual and family theories and practice can be used as different level systems, the application of which can be instituted where there is maximum leverage for change.

REFERENCES

Bloch, D.A. (1976). Including the child in family therapy. In P.J. Guerin (Ed.), *Family Therapy: Theory and Practice*. New York: Gardner Press, pp. 168-181.

Brighton-Cleghorn, J. (1987). Formulations of self and family systems. *Family Process*, 185-201.

Carter, E. & McGoldrick, M. (Eds.) (1980). *The Family Life Cycle: A Framework for Family Therapy*. New York: Gardner Press.

Freud, A. (1981). The concept of developmental lines: Their diagnostic significance. *Psychoanalytic Study of the Child*, 36, 129-137.

Greenberg, J.R. & Mitchell, S.A. (1983). *Object Relations in Psychoanalytic Theory*. Cambridge, Massachusetts: Harvard University Press.

Griff, M.D. (1983). Family play therapy. In K. O'Connor & C. Schaefer (Eds.), *Handbook of Play Therapy*. New York: J. Wiley.

Guerin, P.J. (1976). Family therapy: The first twenty-five years. In P.J. Guerin (Ed.), *Family Therapy: Theory and Practice*. New York: Gardner Press.

Guttman, H.A. (1975). The child's participation in conjoint family therapy. *Journal of the American Academy of Child Psychiatry*, 14, 490-499.

Haley, J. (1973). Strategic therapy when a child is presented as a problem. *Journal of the American Academy of Child Psychiatry*, 12, 641-659.

Harter, S. (1983). Cognitive-developmental conditions in the conduct of play therapy. In K. O'Connor & C. Schaefer (Eds.), *Handbook of Play Therapy*. New York: J. Wiley.

Herschkowitz, S. & Kahn, C. (1980). Toward a psychoanalytic view of family systems. *The Psychoanalytic Review*, (67)1, 45-68.

Katan, A. (1961). Some thoughts about the role of verbalization in early childhood. *Psychoanalytic Study of the Child*, 16, 184-188.

Lerner, S. & Lerner, H. (1983). A systemic approach to resistance: Theoretical and technical considerations. *American Journal of Psychotherapy*, (37)3, 387-399.

McDermott, J.F. & Charles, W.F. (1974). The undeclared war between child and family therapy. *Journal of the American Academy of Child Psychiatry*, 13(3), 422-436.

Nichols, M. (1987). *The Self in the System*. New York: Brunner/Mazel.

Olden, C. (1953). On adult empathy with children. *Psychoanalytic Study of the Child*, 8, 111-126.

Ornstein, A. (1976). Making contact with the inner world of the child: Toward a comprehensive theory of psychoanalytic psychotherapy with children. *Comprehensive Psychiatry*, (17)1, 3-36.

Peller, L. (1954). Libidinal phases, ego development and play. *Psychoanalytic Study of the Child*, 9, 178-198.

Rhodes, S.L. (1977). A developmental approach to the life cycle of the family. *Social Casework*, May, 301-311.

Sager, C.J., Walker, L., Brown, H.S., Crohn, H. & Rodstein, E. (1981). Improving the functioning of the remarried family system. *Journal of Marital and Family Therapy*, January, 3-13.

Sager, C.J., Brown, H.S., Crohn, H., Engel, T., Rodstein, E. & Walker, L. (1983). *Treating the Remarried Family*. New York: Brunner/Mazel.

Samalin, N. (1987). *Loving Your Child Is Not Enough: Positive Discipline that Works*. New York: Viking Penguin.

Satir, V. (1984, revised 1967, original edition 1964). Including the child in family therapy. *Conjoint Family Therapy*. Palo Alto: Science and Behavior Books, 179-206.

Selvini-Palozzoli, M., Cecchin, G., Prata, G. & Boscolo, L. (1978). *Paradox and Counterparadox*. New York: Jason Aronson.

Sluski, C. (1981). Process of symptom production and patterns of symptom maintenance. *Journal of Marital and Family Therapy*, July, 273-280.

Spitz, R. (1975). Life and the dialogue. In H.S. Gaskill (Ed.), *Counterpoint: Libidinal Object and Subject*, 159-174.

Stern, D. (1977). *The First Relationship: Infant and Mother*. Cambridge, Massachusetts: Harvard University Press.

Stierlin, H., Rucker-Embden, I., Wetzel, N., Wirsching, M. (1980). *The First Interview with the Family*. New York: Brunner/Mazel.

Villeneuve, Claude. The specific participation of the child in family therapy. *Journal of the American Academy of Child Psychiatry*, (18)1, 44-53.

von Bertalannfy, L. (1968). *General Systems Theory*. New York: George Braziller.

Watzlawick, P., Beavin, J.H. & Jackson, D. (1967). *Pragmatics of Human Communication: A study of Interactional Patterns, Pathologies, and Paradoxes*. New York: Norton.

Winnicott, D.W. (1971). *Playing and Reality*. Middlesex, England: Penguin.

Zilbach, J.J., Bergel, E.W. & Gass, C. (1972). The role of the young child in family therapy. In C.J. Sager & H.S. Kaplan (Eds.), *Progress in Group and Family Therapy* (pp. 385-400). New York: Brunner/Mazel.

_____ (1986). *Young Children in Family Therapy*. New York: Brunner/Mazel.

An Experiential Family Therapy Training Seminar

Michael Isaiah Bennett
Joan J. Zilbach

We designed a method for teaching clinicians about the treatment of families to overcome certain problems in the approach of our supervisees particularly towards family cases. Supervisees tend to rely on values and techniques derived from their experience with individual psychodynamic psychotherapy, whether as patients or practitioners. Few have been patients themselves in family treatment. The problematic values and techniques include: encouraging the expression of uncomfortable feelings that family members have not agreed to explore; regarding the influence of parents over children as the primary cause of symptoms; concealing clinical information about the child from the parents; and withholding information from family members about the background and opinions of the therapist. In addition, the fact that our supervisees are usually at an earlier stage in their own family life cycles (Zilbach, 1979, 1986, 1988; Carter and McGoldrick, 1980; Combrinck-Graham, 1985; Duvall, 1977) than the parents they see in practice predisposes them to overidentify with the plight of children. Despite their sympathy for children, however, they are often uncomfortable including chil-

Michael Isaiah Bennett, MD, is Director, Adult Emergency and Outpatient Services, Massachusetts Mental Health Center, and Instructor in Psychiatry, Harvard Medical School. Joan J. Zilbach, MD, is affiliated with the Fielding Institute, Santa Barbara, CA and was formerly Consultant, Family Therapy Program, Department of Child Psychiatry, Massachusetts Mental Health Center, Harvard Medical School.

The authors wish to acknowledge the support of Jules Bemporad, MD, the former Director of Child Psychiatric Services at Massachusetts Mental Health Center, as well as suggestions contributed by Peg Dickerman, LICSW.

145

dren in family sessions and fail to gather data about the parent-child interactions (Zilbach, 1986).

SEMINAR DESIGN

We addressed these problems by designing an experiential family therapy training seminar in which participants would be encouraged to reflect on family influences in their own lives. The seminar co-leaders initiated discussions by contributing relevant observations about their own families. They encouraged the discussion of family reminiscences while discouraging the expression of intense personal feelings. The goals included: focusing on normal rather than abnormal behavior; exploring the uniqueness of each family by examining its habits, rituals, traditions and values; ensuring equal sympathy for the dilemmas of parents and children; encouraging an appreciation of the power of families to transmit values and habits and to shape individuals in ways that are often taken for granted; encouraging reflection on the place of the individual in the family life cycle; demonstrating the safety and usefulness of the clinician's discussing his or her own family; and encouraging the inclusion of children in family interviews.

The authors were responsible for family therapy training in the Children's Unit at Massachusetts Mental Health Center, a state hospital and community mental health center run by the Massachusetts Department of Mental Health and affiliated with Harvard Medical School. The family training seminar consisted of 16 biweekly sessions offered to all clinicians interested in family therapy. Interdisciplinary participants (limited to 12) included clinicians with administrative authority over others in the seminar.

During the initial meeting, the leaders explained the seminar's rules: no one was obliged to say anything he or she was not comfortable saying; participants were under no obligation to attend the seminar or to continue attendance; and participants would respect and safeguard the confidentiality of all seminar discussions. The leaders stated that they would ask participants to consider their roles within their own families during the process of the group's discussion and share their observations about their roles in their own families. The leaders then introduced themselves within the context of their own families, e.g., "I am the older of 2 children born to Jewish parents living in the rural West. I am now the father of 1 child, age 2." They emphasized that all readings or intellectual discussions would be considered in the light of the participants' own family history and experiences.

The leaders developed a number of "assignments" to help participants become comfortable and to focus their attention on family issues. These included: requesting participants to introduce themselves to one another by discussing the meaning of their names; requesting participants to describe their position within their family, including family of origin, present family, and extended family; having participants draw pictures of their families or pose other participants in a typical family tableau; and inviting participants to select and play with toys and compare their differing approaches with their early family experiences.

The leaders discovered over time that it was helpful to direct participants to describe and compare the responses of their families to a number of family events and issues. These included: birth order; holidays; religious rituals; family meals; birthdays; births; weddings; work; get-togethers with the extended family; illness and death; discipline of children; response to trauma; economic class; and ethnicity.

The leaders contributed personal reflections about their own families. The goal was to demonstrate that family clinicians can make use of personal material in treatment with safety and comfort, without undermining their special responsibilities as therapists.

PARTICIPANTS' EXPERIENCE

The seminar, which was repeated yearly between 1977 and 1983, seemed to increase participants' awareness of the power and subtlety of family influences on their lives. It deepened their appreciation of the power of ethnicity, religion, nationality, and birth order to shape personality and serve as a focus for therapeutic reflection and increased their ability to tolerate children and childish behavior in settings such as family interviews. (See Kramer, 1984, for a similar group, "TOFG" which had questionnaire evaluation pp. 232-235, and this volume, Kramer, "Perceived Change in Self and

Children Following Participation of a Therapist-Parent in a Therapist's Own Family Group" pp. 173-185.)

The composition of the seminar, which always included people from different stages of the family life cycle, enhanced the ability of participants to understand both sides of the parent-child relationship and trace its development over time. One member, in the late middle stages of the family life cycle, had all her children in college and was helping several members of the previous generation with medical crises; another, in an earlier stage, had all grade school children. Participants included single students and staff members, married individuals considering parenthood, expectant mothers and fathers, parents of infants, school-age children, and children leaving home, and adults caring for ailing parents. Discussions of the parent-child relationship always elicited comments from more than one of these generational stages. Issues included the difficulty in balancing love and limit-setting and the sense of responsibility that parents feel for children in pain and of children for parents in pain. Personal discussions illustrated stages of family development and interactions between individual development and family life cycle.

The seminar's first meeting usually demonstrated two themes: the tendency for participants to take for granted and ignore family frames of reference; and the need for participants to feel safe. The authors demonstrated the first theme by asking participants to note the frame of reference they used to introduce themselves. Initial introductions usually included the participant's name, role as a clinician, and program affiliation within the mental health system. Then the leaders invited participants to identify themselves in terms of their families. After a second round of introductions, many participants realized that they had multiple frames of family reference acquired during different phases of the family life cycle.

Although the amount of personal disclosure was small, participants invariably expressed concern about the degree of safety they would experience in the seminar. Occasionally a participant whose feelings about a family crisis or relationship were intense (e.g., grief after the recent death of a parent) would decide to leave the seminar. The leaders, who supported such decisions, encouraged disclosure of feelings only when participants felt comfortable and urged participants to follow the same policy as family therapists.

The following issues are among the most interesting and typical and often prompted participants to note that they had not been addressed by other didactic seminars or by previous experiences in individual psychotherapy.

Birth Order

Participants with the same birth order were surprised to realize how much they shared in common and derived their style as therapists from their childhood role as helpers within their families. First-borns, who accounted for a disproportionate number of the physicians attending the seminar, recognized in themselves a tendency to help by taking charge and demonstrating expertise, both as children and as adult therapists; clinicians who were younger siblings recognized a tendency to help by encouraging a positive emotional atmosphere without contesting authority. One participant, an oldest child who seemed overbearing as a family therapist, described his family's inability to make decisions without first consulting him.

Holidays

Holidays, especially Thanksgiving and Christmas, evoked affectively intense images that were typical of the varied family styles and issues. Holidays forced many families to reconcile the religious rituals and practices of another country with American practices that were more popular with the younger generation. Often, a family's solution would create conflict with close relatives. Holidays also brought to mind the absence of family members who were excluded, or had excluded themselves, after a conflict. The list of those attending or remaining absent from holiday gatherings was invariably significant, as were the rituals for gathering and including children in festivities.

Names

Names brought forth a wealth of family material: names of which families were proud or ashamed; names changed but still remembered; names bringing an old culture into a new land; surnames carrying forward the identity and values of a member of a previous generation; "real" names in the family's ethnic or religious language; names evoking the protection of a godparent during a coming-of-age ceremony; names for use within the family and names used exclusively at work; maiden names later abandoned, retained, or reclaimed after divorce; nicknames; names that marked one as "different"; names chosen during adulthood; names participants wished to perpetuate; and namings that healed or worsened family conflicts. Often the discussion of names uncovered the participants' sense of who their families wished them to be and how their lives fulfilled family traditions. One participant had acquired, during adult life, two separate names: one, used by colleagues, which identified her within her profession; and the other, used by friends and within her community, which identified her as a wife, mother, and town official. The discussions prompted many participants to inquire further into the reasons behind their parents' choice of their own names.

Family Food Rituals

The authors encouraged reflections about family food and dinner table rituals, including holiday food and meals, and occasionally accentuated these themes by bringing holiday food to the seminar (e.g., Easter eggs, Halloween candy). The consideration of food rituals was an evocative method of drawing information from both children and adults.

Participants noted that their feelings about "being at home" prompted thoughts of dinner table rituals during childhood that had been carried over to their current family life. One participant, who had always shared dinner with both her parents, tolerated her husband's erratic evening work habits until the birth of their first child. Then she discovered how vehemently she desired his attendance at dinner. She was surprised to consider how much these feelings were rooted in her family of origin. Several participants recognized that their feelings about the presence of both parents at an evening meal were so strong that they had never considered other options. Discussions of the family meals also evoked an awareness of ethnic and other differences in family dinner table conversations: loud or quiet; parent- or child-dominated; full of interruptions or polite. Participants became aware of the style and setting of such conversations, apart from their content. One participant noted that changes in family dinners coincided with different phases of the life cycle: she always cooked for her family when her children were younger; later the children shared cooking responsibilities after family discussions of this as a possible change.

Coming to Terms

In the process of considering long-standing and typical family styles and characteristics, seminar participants tended to become somewhat philosophical in accepting painful aspects of family life. This acceptance emerged gradually as participants considered family relationships from a viewpoint other than their own immediate feelings. For instance, after considering her mother as a child and wife in the context of her family's tradition, one participant was able to perceive her mother's rejecting behavior as having powerful causes outside their relationship. As a result, she gradually felt less rejected by her mother and regarded her with less blame and bitterness. Another participant, recalling her inability to mend a family split set off by a disagreement over wedding arrangements, felt less personal responsibility for the problem as she considered the large number of reasons contributing to the split and heard of similar experiences from other, older participants. A participant who had failed to reconcile with her father before his death realized in retrospect that her task had been impossible because of the many family and personal factors blocking their relationship. Participants often observed, with surprise, that it was helpful to review the trauma and limitations of family life from a safe distance.

Personal Contributions from Seminar Leaders

From the outset, participants responded comfortably and constructively to the reflections contributed by the seminar leaders about their own families. For instance, after a participant had discussed his special responsibilities as the oldest child in his family, one of the leaders described some of the similarities and differences she attributed to her role as an only child growing up with an uncle who treated her like a younger sister. On another occasion, the other leader described his role as an interpreter between parents having entirely opposite cognitive and emotional styles. These contributions led seminar participants to additional reflections and demonstrated a way of sharing family material without a feeling of confession or self-exposure. By the end of the year, many participants felt they had acquired a safe method for using their personal experiences in their work as therapists.

The leaders also made use of their disagreements as a focus for reflection and to demonstrate that the airing and resolution of disagreements is a normal and important part of family life. Whether they eventually agreed or continued to disagree, their mutual respect was secure. Their arguments invariably evoked recollections of the different ways parents argued and the factors that made such arguments safe or dangerous.

Family Power

The participation in the seminar of faculty members having administrative power over other participants elicited useful observations about power in family relationships. For instance, some participants noted that their boss, who was present, characteristically avoided giving direct orders. They compared his style to their parents', noting both pros and cons. Their observations prompted him to realize how much he disliked and wished to avoid the dictatorial management style of his own parents. Participants working for one of the seminar leaders noted, without being critical, that his tendency to nag members of his staff about paperwork evoked a variety of responses. He reflected that the pleasure he took in imposing administrative order derived from his dislike of the chaotic and loosely managed household of his childhood.

Estrangements

Every year the subject of family estrangements evoked stories of families irrevocably split by conflict, and the sadness and depression these estrangements caused among family members of multiple generations. Many of the participants felt that their interest in family therapy arose from their wish to heal a split they had experienced in their own families. After such discussions, participants were impressed with the power of such splits to cause pain and impairment and to influence succeeding generations. Helpless to find solutions, they noted that they had learned to live with the pain by limiting their sense of responsibility and achieving a tolerable distance from family members involved in conflict.

Families and Other Systems

As the year progressed, participants applied their observations about roles, rituals, traditions, and relationships in their families to other organizations they encountered, such as schools and inpatient units. For instance, after participants who had suffered a painful year of inpatient residency examined their ward's history and traditions, they realized that in the previous "generation," before they had arrived on the ward, a change in the style and philosophy of the ward's leadership had created the potential for conflict in the "family."

Ethnicity

Participants learned something new about the ethnic uniqueness of family life. For example, one clinician was from India, and his story illustrated the special responsibilities of Indian families for arranged marriages. Another participant was a second generation Irish Catholic. Her description of her father's ties to Ireland revealed the extent to which she had been shaped by the loyalties and moral values of a society from which she was a generation removed.

The conflicts that arise with increasing distance from ethnic heritage were illustrated by a pregnant participant's reflections on her mother's upcoming postnatal visit. Her mother, having traditional Hispanic middle-class values, expected to take over her daughter's household while her daughter spent a prolonged period passively convalescing after childbirth. The daughter, having lived for many years as a self-supporting mental health professional, was accustomed to running her own life and wished to remain in control of her family and her professional life as much as possible. After the birth of her first child, her mother's visit had occasioned considerable conflict. As she reflected on her mother's upcoming visit, older participants described having had similar experiences and coming to the sad realization, as they established their own households, that their values were fundamentally different from those of their parents and that the gulf could never entirely be bridged. The discussion saddened the pregnant participant, but she felt better prepared for her mother's visit.

Family vs. Career

Younger participants contemplating parenthood expressed worries about their ability to balance work and parental responsibilities. They considered how their parents' solution to this issue shaped their own expectations, and how their parents' solution was in turn shaped by previous family traditions, ethnic and religious values and economic realities. Older participants confirmed the realization that the previous generation's experiences and traditions do not always provide a helpful model and that adults of this generation may be obliged to find their own paths and create new traditions.

INFLUENCE OF SEMINAR
ON TREATMENT TECHNIQUE

Seminar members were reluctant to see children together with their families in family treatment. Without the one-to-one attention of individual psychotherapy, children often become disruptive and interrupt adult conversations. In addition, parents become defensive if they are unable to set limits, or if their limit setting appears unduly harsh or leads them to expose angry feelings. In such situations, clinicians find it hard to make parents comfortable, retain control over the interview, and avoid showing displeasure over the parents' response to the child.

Including Children in Family Therapy

The seminar made parent-child interactions more comfortable for participants by encouraging them to understand the dilemmas of parenting. Participants who were parents reflected on the difficulty of balancing love and limit setting and the parent's sense of responsibility for a child's pain. Recollections included: the first time a parent enforced bedtime by letting his 8-month old cry in her crib without taking her out to comfort her; a parent's response to her teen-age son's expulsion from school; a mother's guilt about favoring one child over another; and the helplessness of caring for a sick child. These themes evoked similar feelings from adults caring for their ailing parents.

The seminar demonstrated that simultaneous communication with adults and children is possible, if the clinician is comfortable with play and nonverbal forms of communication. For participants trained as psychodynamic psychotherapists, it was initially upsetting to engage in nonverbal tasks that were potentially revealing and embarrassing, such as choosing toys from a large pile or drawing pictures of one's family. As the leaders elicited comments and observations, however, participants gained confidence in their ability to use such play to gather information without causing embarrassment.

For instance, after being asked to pick toys from a common pile, one participant noted that his concern, while picking out three toys, was that he should not take the best. Another was worried that he would take more than his share. A third worked to fit all the selected toys together. Another worried that he would do less than other participants in the group. These observations illustrated both emotional and cognitive styles, as well as aspects of participants' early family play experiences.

Participants discovered that their play conveyed information, emotion, and individuality without requiring excessive self-exposure. They could turn a serious adult situation into play, and play into adult insight. The language of play was not inferior to adult conversation.

CONCLUSION

In retrospect, seminar participants observed that their training and experience as patients in individual psychotherapy accustomed them to consider the uncovering of feelings as the essence of effective treatment. The seminar engaged them in a process that was meaningful and moving yet did not always require the expression of deeper feelings. One of the leaders, quoting Wordsworth, described the tone of the seminar as "emotion recollected in tranquility." The tone was conversational and descriptive, and the focus was on events, ideas, and family situations that were not necessarily current or immediately painful.

Individual psychotherapy or participation in group therapy training groups had taught seminar members that the deepest insights arise from an examination of transference, dreams, or unconscious feelings. In the seminar, however, they found information of equal value in family stories and descriptions of family rituals. They also were surprised at the amount of information they could learn from drawings and other nonverbal forms of expression. Without devaluing other techniques, the seminar taught the worth of exploring the facts and symbols of family life.

Seminar members expressed surprise that the personal insights and ideas they gained from the seminar had not been considered during their personal individual psychotherapies or psychoanalyses. They concluded that the emotional power of family life may express itself in experiences that often escape the usual assessment techniques of individual psychodynamic psychotherapy. An examination of inner feelings, dreams, or transference may not reveal the importance of motivations that arise from ethnic values or from birth order, for example. Participants realized that human motivation can be more fully understood by using multiple frames of reference, and that one important frame is the individual's place in his or her family.

The seminar leaders' discussion of their own family experiences highlighted therapeutic approaches of which psychodynamically trained clinicians seem unaware. According to psychodynamic theorists, the clinician should withhold personal information in order to encourage the development in the patient of transference feelings, which then provide a useful subject for examination. Clinicians learned in the seminar that withholding personal information may undermine a tentative alliance, and that the clinician may legitimately choose the opposite approach: i.e., to promote a positive alliance by presenting more of the "real self." In addition, the clinician's willingness to discuss his or her family may put patients at ease by demonstrating that painful family subjects may be discussed without excessive self-exposure or embarrassment.

There are a number of possible reasons for the seminar's ability to discourage participants from overidentifying with children as the victims of parents. These include: the encouragement of a multigenerational perspective; the uncovering of causal factors within the family over which parents had little control; and the inclusion in the seminar of the viewpoints of participants, including the seminar leaders, with varying degrees of administrative power. In effect, by including these viewpoints the seminar encouraged those with less power to identify with and understand the helplessness of those who appear to have more power and vice versa.

A family seminar like the one we have described enacts the principles that we believe are essential for good family treatment: to respect the family's right to privacy; to take responsibility for setting rules and creating an emotional climate that makes the family feel comfortable; to understand and use the rich variety of assessment techniques that elicit family data; and to use their own personalities and family experiences to set a safe course for the family's examination of itself within the family treatment.

REFERENCES

Carter, E.A. and McGoldrick, M. (1980). The Family Life Cycle and Family Therapy: An Overview. In: Carter, E. and McGoldrick, M. (Eds.), *The Family Life Cycle*, pp. 3-19. New York: Gardner Press.

Combrinck-Graham, L. (1985). A Developmental Model for Family Systems. *Family Process*, 24: 139-151.

Duvall, E. (1977). *Marriage and Family Development*, 5th Edition. Philadelphia: Lippincott.

Kramer, J. (1984). *Family Interfaces: Transgenerational Patterns*, pp. 231-250. New York: Brunner/Mazel.

Zilbach, J.J. (1979). Family Development and Familial Factors in Etiology. In: Noshpitz, J. (Ed.), *Basic Handbook of Child Psychiatry*, Vol. 2, pp. 62-87. New York: Basic Books.

Zilbach, J.J. (1986). *Young Children in Family Therapy*. New York: Brunner/Mazel.

Zilbach, J.J. (1988). The Family Life Cycle: A Framework for Understanding Children in Family Therapy. In: Combrinck-Graham, L. (Ed.), *Children in Families* pp. 46-66. New York: Guilford.

Play with Young Children in Family Therapy: An Extension of the Therapist's Holding Capacity

Jill Savege Scharff

PLAY: AN ASPECT OF THE THERAPIST'S HOLDING CAPACITY

In family therapy, the therapist's task is to provide a helpful environment in which the whole family can participate and which it can shape according to its unique expressions of need, thought and feeling. The environment derives from the design of the office, from the way arrangements for consultation and therapy are handled, and from the ability to listen thoughtfully, to engage, to be affected, to tolerate anxiety, to reflect upon experience, and to communicate understanding intent. This ability has been called the therapist's "contextual holding capacity" (Scharff and Scharff, 1987). Through this, the therapist provides the context for expression of the family's usual patterns of relating which derive from the complex interaction of present relationships and previous experience with significant others in the family of origin and in the present family during earlier periods of development.

The first step in creating the context is to communicate the expectation of seeing the whole family. To offer "whole family understanding" (Zilbach, 1986), the therapist needs the whole family at the session. When that family includes a crying baby or a messy toddler or an unstoppable three-year old, then the context must accommodate to their needs if the family is to feel fully held in the therapist's mind. This is where play comes in. Therapists need to be able to play with families that have young children. The contextual holding capacity has to include comfort with play — and the accompanying noise, mess, and regression, all common features of ordinary family life.

This sounds so obvious, it is a surprise to discover that it needs saying. It seems strange that a family therapist might not think of very young children as part of the family to be seen in treatment. But it is understandable that family therapists trained only to work with adults and adolescents might be reluctant to include younger children in family therapy. Some of them deal with this by referring the case to a child and family therapist. Unfortunately, some will exclude children under 13 so as to reduce the family to suit their skills because they have not had experience with child psychotherapy. Then the family, its younger children, and the therapist lose an opportunity. The family cannot express its total experience, the young children are discriminated against, and the therapist cannot get whole family understanding to share with the family.

Therapists who are child-trained often specialize in individual play therapy and have not been trained in family work. Furthermore, references to working with young children in family therapy in the literature are few and far between. So, many a therapist has been uninformed about play in family therapy until recently (Scharff and Scharff, 1987; Zilbach, 1986).

PROVISION OF THE PLAY SPACE

The family therapist needs an office big enough to allow for six to eight seats and floor or table space to play on. It is best if the play space is in the middle of the circle of chairs so that it is easy for grown-ups and therapist to watch or play while still talking. If the play space is at the end of the room or in the corner, this may give a "go away and play" message which devalues the play. Play is not a diversion; it is central to the work of family therapy with children.

I suggest just a few toys so that the child is not overwhelmed with choices. Paper and a set of crayons and markers can be used by all ages, although some mothers for good reason prefer the markers to be out of toddlers' reach. Blocks are basic and require a few animals and vehicles to expand their usefulness for four-year olds and other children. I generally stop there when I am packing a bag for doing a teaching interview. But in my office I also like to have large paper, small black-skinned and white-skinned doll family characters, a regular size doll and doll bed, and some puppets. Lego is fun for older children, but again the smaller pieces should not be used with infants around. I do not use any board games because I prefer to work with fantasy play, but I have supervised a student who made surprisingly good use of them in family therapy.

These selections offer a range of media for self-expression and give the message that the family can have fun while working on serious issues. Thus the provision of play materials creates a play space which reflects an inner readiness on the part of the therapist to engage in play.

In family therapy the grown-ups sit talking while the children are playing, a grown-up sometimes joining the children on the floor or perhaps intervening in a dispute over a toy. A microcosm of the at home situation is reproduced in the office. We can observe how the parents support or suppress the play, how they manage sibling rivalry, and how they communicate to their children. The therapist models an interested but nonintrusive method of following and exploring the themes shown in the play so that the children's contribution is included. At the same time the parents learn how to listen to their children at play, which improves the parents' holding capacity for the family.

HOW PLAY WORKS

Play is the natural vehicle for expression of the young child, as the child moves, jumps, or crawls around the room with the toys. The child expresses ideas and feelings symbolically in the safety of displacement onto the toy characters or general play media. The importance of motoric expression should not be minimized; for the child who has to sit on his needs for physical release will hold back other aspects of himself too. Both motoric and symbolic routes of expression are important in the reduction of anxiety and thereby facilitate the child's comfort at the session. Play also offers the therapist who can follow its message an elaboration of the unconscious themes of the family — including its unconscious transference to the therapist — often long before these are expressed verbally by the adults. Play can be taken as a gloss on the verbal themes, a confirmation of understanding, or may actually lead the way to direct discussion of the family issues and conflicts expressed in displacement through the play.

Play may be more or less central to the family work from one session to another. The character of the play varies depending on the ages of the children and the number of them playing. For instance, in the toddler's family the play will not be clearly thematic, but will demonstrate problems of sharing, messing, destroying, getting into things, going to the bathroom, and needing support and discipline from parents whereas in the family of the latency child, the play will be more symbolic and less action-oriented. Adolescents may play with their sneakers, tear at holes in their jeans, shred tissue, or twist hair in addition to scribbling or sketching while talking. The importance of play varies from one family to another both in the same family and even in the therapist who just cannot take it in as well at some times as at others. The therapist's countertransference is essential to understanding the play, especially when the themes are obscured by dense displacement or by blocks to comprehension in the therapist.

As different play reflects varying degrees of displacement from the source of the conflict, so the therapist's response to play varies from simple observation without comment to full interpretation. Between those extremes, the therapist may silently analyze his or her response to the play, ask about the play, intervene through the play or use the play as a metaphor to illustrate the family's spoken theme. Play may introduce new themes. Play may be a safe area in which to offer interpretation about conflict, relationships, and underlying anxiety. Then comes the work of reconstruction, linking the insights from play to family living and then watching the next piece of play in reaction to interpretation.

PLAY IN A DIAGNOSTIC CONSULTATION

The following example, taken from two diagnostic sessions that have been recorded on videotape, illustrates these varying uses of play in family therapy with very young children. It also shows the usefulness of a co-therapy model in that situation.

Mrs. W. complained to a clinic social worker that her overactive sixteen-month-old Brooke was into everything and exhausting her. She admitted that Terri, her four-year old, was also demanding. When frustrated, Terri threw temper tantrums and refused to listen to reason. Because Mrs. W. suffered from severe unremitting migraine headaches for the last two months of her second pregnancy during which she took codeine frequently, her baby went through withdrawal after delivery. She was guilty and worried that "being born an addict" had damaged this child so that now she cried too much. And her husband came home at the end of the day, criticizing her management of both children and asking why the toys were not picked up. She felt bombarded by all of them.

The social worker arranged for a family evaluation by her consultant, Dr. David Scharff [*DES*] and me. Incidentally, although we teach together and have written together, he and I usually work alone, but this social worker was interested in having us use a co-therapy model for teaching and so referred to both of us.

The W.s arrived with beautifully dressed children. Mother deftly moved our magic markers out of reach. Immediately baby Brooke started screaming. Mother offered a crayon which was rejected and a pacifier which stopped the yell. Four-year-old Terri settled to play purposefully with the crayons, producing a drawing which the baby then scribbled on until she was pushed away. Every time Brooke was thwarted she opened her mouth and yelled until Dad or Mom placated her with pacifier or bottle. Her mouth gaped like a big dark hole, her grief never more than temporarily assuaged.

Mother explained, as she gave the screaming child her pacifier, that Brooke was born addicted to codeine and had to go through withdrawal. "I was up every hour with that fretful baby the first few months," she told us. "Even now," she added, "If I leave the room, Brooke cries." As if to prove her mother wrong, Brooke calmly walked away and handed a doll baby to DES and enjoyed with him a game of handing the baby back and forth. Mother in surprise cried, "She's not clinging to me here!" [*I thought there was a trace of unconscious outrage and disappointment in her tone.*] Father said, "I just leave Brooke to cry. Why can't my wife do that?" Mother complained, "It's not possible. She cries more for me than for you." [*I noted some pride in Mother's remark. I had a sense of parental competition, Mother claiming ownership of the cry as a proof of love and Father achieving extinction of the cry as a proof of competence.*]

Right on key, Brooke began to cry and was settled with a bottle while Terri, playing with puppets, had the horse and rabbit fight about which of them had the crayon first. Meanwhile the parents were talking about Father's need for a well-balanced checkbook and a tidy house and Mother's inability to keep the house or the checkbook because of all the errands to do and messes to clean up. Then Terri tried to draw a picture for DES but could not get it done because Brooke messed on it. [**Here the play reflected the theme, as the sibling play picked up Mother's complaint of mess and interruption.**] Mother continued, "I can't get everything done. I'm exhausted because Brooke gets me up five times a night." Brooke had found a toy garbage can with a pop-up Oscar-the-Grouch inside. She was playing at popping open and shutting the lid. Then she took it to her Dad.

[I was thinking of referring to Brooke's portrayal of Mother as a grouch, but I thought that this might be too hurtful to Mother. More important to me was the "now-you-see-him-now-you-don't" quality of the play which I thought was a re-creation of Brooke's nighttime reunions with and leave-takings from Mother. Her playful repetition indicated an attempt to work in the displacement on the conflict over separation. Brooke, in handing Father the pop-up toy, was looking to him to validate her struggle. I was thinking that Brooke was indicating her readiness to be more separate if and when her parents would forego the gratification to their guilt that her clinging afforded.]

So to them I said, "It's hard for you to see Brooke through her period of frustration because you cannot bear the guilty feelings of seeing her suffer any more than she already did. I also think it's hard for you to admit how angry you are at her for all the suffering she has caused you."

"Well, I know I'm angry and that's why I put her in her room — otherwise I'd hit her," said Father, while Mother looked disapprovingly at him.

The parents continued to discuss their complaints against each other and how these arose from the conflict between his mid-West immigrant ethic and her California laid-back style. Father became extremely critical of Mother and Brooke climbed on Mother's lap and looked concerned while Father laughed and Mother jokingly patted his arm. I said, "You feel you have to laugh off angry feelings, but Brooke is aware of Mom's upset and her need for comfort." The parents responded by getting angrier. Terri created a diversion by painting all her toenails with purple marker. And Brooke started to cry to get someone to take off her shoes, too.

In this summarized example I have not reported in full the number of times Brooke began to cry. But in the session, when I found myself counting them, I knew I was defending against the pain by quantifying it. When she cried, her mouth became a gaping, black hole, taking over her face while her shriek cut through to me tearing at my chest. The cries of children other than my own do not usually effect me intensely, but this cry had enormous power to evoke pain and helplessness. Then I realized this was true for me only at the beginning of the cry which began petering out even before the bottle was offered. And many times Brooke merely played with the bottle, pushing the nipple in and out. My countertransference response gelled with my detection of the game of peek-a-boo with the nipple as well as with the pop-up Oscar-the-Grouch garbage can.

This analysis enabled me to question the parents with empathy and yet distance about their experience of the cry. They too had wondered if Brooke might not keep it up if not gratified by Mother. After we worked through their defenses against guilt and anger at Brooke and after I showed them the evidence of her readiness, they agreed to try to let her cry it out.

The family was unable merely to hold the baby and allow her to quiet herself. It was painful to listen to her scream and watch her being fed when not hungry or see her aching mouth plugged with a pacifier. Because of guilt and anger, this family had a deficient holding capacity for a family member who needed to express helplessness, rage, and fear at separation. The family in this situation was afraid that the therapist would be similarly deficient. This has been called the family's transference to our holding capacity (Scharff and Scharff, 1987). It emerged in phone calls before and after the session, checking the arrangements, and worrying that videotape might be used in a way that would cause suffering to them.

In the second diagnostic session a week later, the parents returned to the theme of their upset over Mother's failure to run a perfect house. Mother spoke of missing her mother to whom she used to turn for advice and help. Meanwhile Brooke was sitting on Mother's lap sucking on her pacifier while Terri built a low, enclosed building with two sheep inside and Oscar-the-Grouch coming outside. [*I noticed that, as usual, Terri played contentedly and unobtrusively. She made the sort of low, enclosed building typical of four-year-old girls and her use of animals was also age-appropriate. I was wondering if the two sheep represented the parents from whom the Grouch—representing Terri or Brooke—was separating, or if the two sheep represented the identification between Mother and baby and Oscar represented the growing child that differentiates from the symbiosis. There was not enough evidence to be sure.*]

As Mother and Father spoke more heatedly about their differences, Brooke messed up Terri's game. Terri punched her. Brooke started crying and returned to Mother's lap. DES said that when the parents were talking about their difficulties, Brooke and Terri had fought to draw anger on to themselves. "I think it's their way of trying to bust up the fight," he added, "Because it happens when you are talking about your anger at each other." "No! It's **any** time we talk, they fight," Mother corrected him.

Father went on to describe Terri's insistence on being heard and on interrupting her parents' conversation. I said "So Terri wants to bust up Mother's and Father's being together, as well as Mother's and Brooke's closeness." Terri responded in play: she had Oscar-the-Grouch peek out at some cows who wanted to play with him. "He's wondering what they're doing," she explained.

[**This play at the surface level mirrors Terri's distrust of her parents' interest in her. It also suggests her oedipal concerns about dealing with exclusion by curiosity and wanting to watch. Now that these two levels of play had become apparent, I could see the fighting as having to do with a struggle about which developmental level would dominate. Would Terri regress to Brooke's level or could Brooke advance to Terri's?**] At this point, the girls began to play in parallel with no conflict, Brooke putting dolls in cars and saying bye-bye to them and Terri developing her animal play to include their getting on each other's backs.

[Here the family is able to allow differentiation of individual needs for expression — Brooke to express preoedipal separation themes and Terri to explore oedipal concerns about exclusion, inclusion, and now more obviously sexuality.]

Momentarily, we were able to talk of the children's envy of the parents' time together. But as we did, Terri again pushed Brooke off the game and again Brooke cried. Mother took Brooke on her lap and told Terri that she knew it was upsetting to have Brooke spoiling things, but she must not punch her. Mother said that she and her husband had read that a four-year old could be expected to be angry at a new baby. "So," she went on, "We were both very sensitive to Brooke's anger and did lots of things special for her, but she did not respond." [Obviously, Mother meant to say she had been sensitive to Terri's anger.] I said that Mother's slip suggests that she *is* preoccupied with Brooke—which Terri has picked up. Mother took my comment as a correction rather than an interpretation and went on describing, now using the correct name, how much Father still does with Terri who is nonetheless jealous and says, "All you care about is Brooke."

Meanwhile in play, Terri had Oscar let the sheep out because he was lonely and wanted to play with them. **[Here the play seems to be focused at the preoedipal level of wanting to be part of the mother-infant couple.]** So I said, "You can do so much for Terri as a four-year old now. But you can never make her your baby again. That's what she's jealous about." "Well, yes," said Mother thoughtfully. "She will come to me and say 'Wa-wa hold me.' Maybe she wants to be a baby again." "Not a baby," I retorted, "*the* baby."

Now Terri was offensively guarding her play, fearing Brooke would try to knock it down and Brooke, crying, went back to Mother. I commented on how Brooke's piercing cry was used to cement herself to Mother. "Exactly!" said Mother. "I can't even take a shower in peace. As soon as I get out of the shower, I hear her crying . . ." Immediately Brooke cried for no apparent reason and clung to Mother who had to interrupt her example to talk soothingly to Brooke and then returned to her story to say that Terri didn't ever cry like that.

[Here is a re-enactment in the session of a typical frustration sequence at home. Of course, this a common complaint by the mother of a toddler, but two items distinguish it from normal:

1. The mother continues to take a shower when no one else is there to mind the toddler.
2. This toddler's cry is more wrenching than most.

(Incidentally, as an aside, many a mother solves the problem by taking the toddler into the shower with her, which also has behavioral and emotional consequences.)]

Mother went on to describe that she gets mad at Terri, too. "Still," she said, "I don't yell. I just explain that I don't like what Terri did and then I give her a hug. Then Terri says, 'I'm bad. You think I'm bad and I hate you.'" And at this, Mother added, "I get even more mad. I don't know where she learned it. We never say she is bad. We never say, 'I hate you.' we say, 'I don't like what you did, but I love you.'"

"That is the sort of advice to teachers and parents that sounds good," I agreed, "But surely only teachers can follow it all the time." Mother replied, "Yes, I am a teacher and it works well in the classroom." DES pointed out that Terri was nonetheless registering Mother's disapproval. Mother anxiously interrupted, "But we always follow criticism with affection so she won't feel bad." DES asked, "So *who* won't feel bad?" Mother looked shocked, Father nodded gravely, and DES asked about how the parents had felt when criticized as children.

[Here DES was taking an object relations history at a moment of affect. No formal history was taken, no genogram done, because these yield facts without linkage to the present interaction. He asked the question at a point when the history was alive in the session, recreated in the present relationships.]

Father gave many graphic examples of not being good enough for his mother who held grudges against him for every misdemeanor. I could see how he had become openly critical, blunt, and forthright so as not to be a pent-up, resentful person like his mother, but I could also see how he projected into his wife an aspect of himself that his mother felt to be not good enough. His wife, in contrast, did not want to hurt people by direct criticism and went to such lengths to be tactful and positive that she was left, not unlike her husband's mother, with a store of resentment.

Now near the end of the second session, Mother told of her growing up. Her sister had been blunt like her husband and had become manic-depressive. Any small comment could set her off, so Mrs. W. learned to tiptoe around her feelings. She tended to do the same with her children and her husband, a courtesy he, at least, did not require. As Mother told this, Terri and Brooke began to fight again and Father said, "Is your sister pickin' on you again?"

[Here is an example of sibling strain being discussed among one generation, being described as it recurs in the marital relationship through projective identification, and being enacted in the next generation through play in the session.]

Brooke was comforted and then went off to lie in the doll bed, very still. Mother talked of her own mother as her best chum, out doing things as girls together while father stayed to work in the yard. I could not make sense of Brooke's corpse-like play until Mother said that her father had died working in his yard when she was 19. She was angry at him for allowing his perfectionism to drive him to an early death. Terri meanwhile was playing with the animals, telling DES, "The horse is lonely, but the two sheep are not lonely 'cos they got each other." **[Here the same play that was earlier understood only to be about the child's exclusion from the parents now has the additional meaning of Mother and her sister missing their dead father or of Mother and her mother missing Father who stayed in the yard while they went out.]** DES interpreted that it seemed important to Mother to not do things perfectly because her father's perfectionism took him away from her and her mother, intensifying their need for each other, and ultimately killing him. He went on, "Now Mother worries that being compulsive will take her away from the children and Father worries that not being compulsive will take her away from him. Instead, Mother is compulsive about never getting angry at her naughty and messy children just as she tried not to be mad at her father for dying."

That the information about Mother's father's death came up near the end of the session was unconsciously determined by their problems with separation and loss, which were probably aggravated by the family's reaction to completing the diagnostic phase and not knowing whether they would be taken on in therapy or would be referred and thus lose one or both of the co-therapy team. It is also often found that affect-laden material comes up at the end of the session because of the protection afforded by there being too little time to explore it thoroughly.

TRANSFERENCE AND COUNTERTRANSFERENCE IN CO-THERAPY

The therapist becomes aware of feelings and reactions to the family group. These constitute the countertransference. Once the therapist separates off responses unique to his or her own personality, the persisting feelings specific to this family then offer evidence about the family's inner relationships and fantasies that determine how it relates to others. In co-therapy, the reception of the family's inner object relations occurs mainly within the co-therapy relationship. Often there will be a splitting of family qualities experienced as residing in one and the other therapist. This gives a further example, usefully displaced away from the primary family relationships, which reflects the way the family has assigned attributes to its various members who then embody and enact the basic family conflict. The co-therapy relationship provides an exceptionally useful culture medium because it is open to process and review by both therapists. Their relationship becomes a subject for study by family and therapists in order to shed light on the family patterns of relating.

In this situation, I was experiencing some tension between DES and myself in which I felt he was taking control, talking too much, and oblivious to my contributions. But when I reviewed his actual behavior I could not justify my feeling. It was time to scrutinize my countertransference.

I was feeling put down by my more talkative co-therapist husband. I felt he had more authority than I had and I felt ignored by the family except when Mother caught my eye in a meaningful female-to-female glance as she described her awful man or child. I concluded that I was experiencing in the transference some of the denigration of the woman's role that Mother felt. I found myself envying my co-therapist's ease with play yet I was becoming more and more dissatisfied with my work and his. We did not seem to be a cooperative team. And I could not find a way to say any of this. I examined this feeling, reviewed the reality bases for it, and concluded that I was receiving in the co-therapy relationship the projection from the couple of a transference to us from their relationship that derived from the previous generation. I, as Mrs. W.'s father, felt remote, and then in danger of being killed off if I did not fight. As her mother, I felt pulled into being a buddy with her. As Father's mother criticising him, I was feeling that my co-therapist was not good enough. As Mr. W. himself, I was feeling that my spouse's work was not good enough. Like Terri I was feeling interrupted and like Brooke I could not find words for my discomfort.

Without more information about Mr. W.'s father, I could not quite complete this preliminary object relations history as experienced in the countertransference. Nonetheless, by this point in the assessment, this countertransference analysis helped me to appreciate the transgenerational transmission of the object relations into the marriage and then beyond into Terri who felt so bad and into Brooke whose scream had to be suppressed. These projections from the parents seemed to represent the blackness, emptiness, and agony of the combined families of origin experienced in separation from the attentive mother and from the withdrawn and ultimately dead father.

After the diagnostic session, DES and I reviewed our countertransference which had been experienced most acutely in me, just as in the couple Mrs. W. felt the most pain. After metabolizing our reactions, he and I would be free to work with these projections into our relationship during ongoing therapy. In this case, however, as in so many others, the family could not afford two therapists. So ongoing co-therapy analysis could not be done, but the experience was registered and used to understand future responses of the therapist working alone.

This family accepted a recommendation for conjoint couple and family therapy with me, but not until it was reestablished that indeed I, too, was a trained child and family psychiatrist. Throughout the interview, it emerged, they had thought I was there "as his wife." My countertransference response of denigration was now clarified and provided a basis for my future work with the family.

In summary, comfort with play is an extension of the therapist's holding capacity. The therapist who can respond to play as a communication facilitates the recreation of the child's view of family life. The attitude of providing for, encouraging, and valuing play communicates interest in the children and in the forgotten childhood of the parents and sets the stage for creative, playful, yet serious work on family issues.

REFERENCES

Scharff, D.E. and Scharff, J.S. (1987). Object Relations Family Therapy. New York: Jason Aronson.

Zilbach, J.J. (1986). *Young Children in Family Therapy*. New York: Brunner/Mazel.

Perceived Change in Self
and Children Following Participation
of a Therapist-Parent
in a Therapist's Own Family Group

Jeannette R. Kramer

I have been leading Therapist's Own Family Groups (T.O.F.G.) since 1977. These training seminars, while based on Bowen theory, use a multifaceted approach. Both discussion and group process are included, in addition to family diagraming and occasional sculpting, roleplaying, and rehearsal. Most of the therapist-trainees develop plans for changing themselves with their original family members and many begin to put these changes into effect during the training period.

I have consistently used two different formats. One is a 20-hour Seminar in the Center's* Short Term Program Series, meeting for 4 hours once a month for 5 months, with 4 to 8 therapists per group. The other format is a 12-hour Preceptor Group of 5 or 6 therapists which meets for 2 hours every other week for 6 sessions during a quarter in the Center's Two Year Training Program. Although the 12-hour groups are shorter, students have already attended 8 hours of classes in which I have presented theory, techniques, and videotaped examples from my own and client families.

The participants fill out questionnaires following each seminar.

Jeanette R. Kramer, Staff and Faculty of the Center for Family Studies/The Family Institute of Chicago.

---

*Center for Family Studies/The Family Institute of Chicago, Institute of Psychiatry, Northwestern Memorial Hospital and Northwestern University Medical School, Chicago, IL.

173

Although there is no specific focus on nuclear family and it was not addressed directly in the group, the questionnaire asks not only about changes with family of origin, but also about changes in nuclear family members. Since I was engaged in the supervision of family therapists and also in the treatment of families including children, I had become interested in the children of family therapists in training. The literature contains only a few references to young children in family therapy (Ackerman, 1970, Bergel, Gass and Zilbach, 1968, Bloch, 1976, Chasin, 1981, Dowling and Jones, 1978, Zilbach, Bergel and Gass, 1972, Zilbach, 1982, 1986). There are no references to children of family therapists in training, and I became curious about this.

Many of the therapists, working in a variety of ways, wrote powerfully about changes in themselves as they worked with their own families. The quotations which follow are taken from the following areas of the questionnaires and specifically include their comments about changes with their own children.

1. Goals and issues
2. Other accomplishments not listed as goals and issues
3. The most significant event in the group and the cause of its significance
4. Changes with family of origin members and their impact
5. Changes with nuclear family members and their impact
6. Changes with client families

#1 FEMALE THERAPIST

"The most significant event (in the T.O.F.G.) was roleplaying myself as a child with my younger sister and family of origin and then roleplaying myself with my son and the rest of my nuclear family. Although I had had an intellectual understanding of my transfer of feelings of being 'crowded' and clung to and bothered from my younger sister to my oldest child, the roleplay made me viscerally aware of my feelings, how angry and helpless I felt, and how much I confused the two relationships. Both relationships have subsequently greatly improved" (*Family Interfaces: Transgenerational Patterns*, Jeannette R. Kramer, Brunner/Mazel, 1985. p. 317).

"With my son I have learned to identify some of my irritation with him as a transference of feeling from my relationship with my younger sister. I feel relief at understanding my feelings."

"With Mother, I am de-triangling, talking to her alone about us, asking for and developing a more individuated relationship with her."

"With my sister I am doing the same as with Mother, plus some work on sharing feelings of my having felt crowded by her when growing up and her having sensed my irritation but never knowing why. We are closer and more relaxed."

#2 FEMALE THERAPIST

"The most significant event was when the leader told me to examine the pattern of male and female relationships in my family. It was significant because I recognized why the women grew up to be independent and competent while the men grew up to be passive and alcoholic. With this insight, I examined the way I treated my son and daughter and changed some of our interactions. I'm giving my son more age-appropriate responsibilities."

"With my 7-year-old son, I am allowing him to make age-appropriate decisions instead of being overprotective, because I don't want him to grow up to be passive, with a low self-esteem. The impact has been very positive since there has been a decrease in conflict between him and his younger sister. He feels more responsible and older than his sister and this has increased his self-esteem."

"With my mother I have decreased my mediator role and feel this has de-triangled me from my mother with other family members. My mother has begun to deal with family members directly instead of going through me to them."

"With my father, instead of giving more time and attention to my mother, I have attempted to increase my behavior with my father. He is less on the periphery and is quite talkative if I give him the individual attention. I feel that my mom criticizes my dad less in our conversation since I have included him when I visit their house.''

#3 FEMALE THERAPIST

"The most significant event was the result of something a group member said. I realized over the next month that I was stuck and had to take control of my life again. The power of one person's work on another in the group surprised me and stays with me when I think of the group's impact. It was significant because the structure of our nuclear family changed for the better. I began to move and so did my 6-year-old daughter. It was very moving to see her drawings free up after 2 years. We began to heal after a difficult, painful 3 years of losses.''

"With my oldest daughter, I'm more aware of her sensitivity to me; I'm helping her feel less responsible for my bad days. She's less dependent on me, less angry at me. We are beginning to enjoy each other as we did during her early years (she is no longer enuretic and her childhood asthma has diminished markedly). There is more trust and acceptance for both of us.''

"With my mother there is less need to take care of her. I am understanding her earlier poor 'mothering' of me better. I am amazed at changes in our relationship. I'm beginning to see how difficult her choices were and to let go of years of frustration and anger towards her. We are enjoying each other for the first time I can remember.''

"With my youngest daughter (3 years), I have more time for her and am able to give her more affection and attention. Very special for both of us.''

#4 FEMALE THERAPIST

"The most significant part was the recognition that I need to work on my relationship with my only brother and also a beginning understanding of some things I can do to effect this. It was significant because of my recognition that there is 'unfinished business' between the two of us which has a negative effect on the way I treat my youngest son and which hinders my effectiveness with certain client families that are similar to my family of origin."

"With my brother, it is important for me not to see him as the victim or to feel excessively 'sorry' for him. This has direct impact on how I treat my own children and in the families I see where there is a markedly 'dysfunctional' family member. I had related to him as if he were about 13 years old before the seminar. It is very difficult because it is painful to get to know him as an adult. I am saddened by his wasted life and the sadness he feels about how his life has been. I am hopeful that my effort with my brother will help me to be a better mother to both my sons, now 10 and 12. I am aware I am very afraid I'll make mistakes with them that will impede their individuality and maturing."

"With my oldest son, now that he is entering adolescence, I need to let him find his own way and to fail, if necessary, at 12 so he can succeed at age 21. With my youngest son I need to continue to be aware of the importance of letting go and allowing him to be himself and to fail, if necessary."

"With my mother, I am trying to do detriangling with her vis à vis my brother and father. I appreciate how easy it is to get sucked into triangular situations."

#5 MALE THERAPIST

"The most significant event was an empty chair exercise the leader used to help me re-create a conversation with my father before he died in which he distanced himself from me and I had felt helpless to bridge the gap and get closer to him. In that conversation, my father had congratulated me on an academic award, then pointed out how my intelligence made me resemble my mother more than I resembled him; in the same breath he exclaimed how difficult it was for my mother and him to communicate with each other. The empty chair exercise helped me to realize how the encounter with my father (and other encounters like it) could have had a different outcome; how I shared responsibility for its outcome (rather than just being a victim of my father's withdrawal) and how I might handle such isolation in current life situations. Though I don't want to exaggerate the impact of that one exercise, it had lasting effects.''

"I used the seminar primarily to examine issues of father as emotional outsider in the family process. Simultaneously, however, I'm involving myself in my son's life in new ways. This was a decision my wife and I were making, but being in the seminar helped me develop new ways of talking to both my kids. They both also became more outspoken in making emotional demands on me during the past few months" (*Family Interfaces: Transgenerational Patterns*, Jeannette R. Kramer, Brunner/Mazel, 1985. p. 314-315).

#6 FEMALE THERAPIST

"The most significant event was talking to my father in an empty chair and realizing, with the leader's help, that I wanted him to change his past way of behaving and make it different and seeing this as an unrealistic and unfulfillable unfair goal. It was significant because I didn't know I felt that way and wanted him to change what he *had done* so long ago. Now I think I can approach him more realistically and acceptingly and maybe communicate better because I won't be trying to get him to change the past.''

"With my father I have thought a lot about my unfinished angers and hurts vis-à-vis him and hope to talk more openly and usefully with him and somehow work out my own acceptance of who he is more thoroughly.''

"With my mother I feel newly angry at her for deprivation of affection and tenderness as I see its negative effects as I try to relate to my daughters. I don't know if this is a step forward or backward.''

"With my oldest daughter I am clearer about the need to set clear, simple limits on her behavior, use pat formulas and phrases if necessary, and not engage in long conversations, explanations, and arguments with her. I see that guilt keeps me relating to her in situations where walking away would be more caring.''

"With my youngest daughter I see that she is as needy as my eldest of support and also of clear, non-wordy limits and that she has her self-doubts, too, and I shouldn't idealize her so."

"With client families I identified with rebellious teenagers and not with parents. Now I see myself as the adult and can identify more with adults and less with kids—which is growth for me" (*Family Interfaces*, p. 324).

#7 FEMALE THERAPIST

"My biggest accomplishment was 'getting it all together'—my acceptance of my family which allowed for acceptance of myself. Integrating who I am; where I started and where I am at times seemed to me to be an impossible chasm to bridge."

"The most significant event was the empty chair work the leader did with me in the final session—with me before I was married, then in my first marriage, and in my second marriage. It was significant because it has been helpful in developing a sense of unity—bridging where I started and where I am now in my life."

"With my mother, I am aware of how she would set me up for arguments. She would become angry at another family member, would not confront them, but instead explode with me. In the past I have interacted with her by igniting. I have been focusing back on who she is having the argument with and refusing to accept it as my problem. I am having a sense of feeling better about my boundary issues."

"With my son I have been able to greatly diminish my protectiveness of him. It has allowed him more growth room and has certainly helped me to be less anxious."

#8 MALE THERAPIST

"The most significant event the leader's confrontation of my wish that my father would change and her assurance that *I* had the power to change unrelated to his permission, acceptance, or willingness. It was significant because it focused on my reluctance (resistance) to making unilateral changes on my own initiative. The challenge encouraged me to do so."

"With my father I am coming to recognize that I do not *need* his approval which enables me to deal with him more as he is and less like I would like him to be."

"I am insisting less that my son deal with me only on my terms. He is 14 years old and we are talking about how the next few years will be difficult for our relationship."

#9 MALE THERAPIST

"The most significant event was sculpting my family of origin. It was emotionally powerful, providing perceptions and linkages that I had not known before and an opportunity to evaluate my role in terms of family patterns."

"Since then I have been closer and less conflictual with my father and I am more assertive with my mother and treat her less gingerly."

"With my son I have learned to not always be so involved and to appropriately move away and permit him to differentiate."

The sculpture also had impact on his actions with client families. He wrote:

"In the family of origin sculpture I realized the powerful confronting position I had in my family (not a victim), and suddenly began seeing adolescents as having too much control and parents not enough. If I sense myself getting into a battle with a parent for control, now I back off; before I would move ahead" (*Family Interfaces*, p. 318).

#10 FEMALE THERAPIST

"The most significant event was work that I did in the group re: my emotional turmoil that resulted from my husband's receiving a promotion, including my fear of loss of my sisters' love if I told them. After rehearsing in the group, I was able to tell my sisters clearly and simply about my husband's promotion without hedging or disqualifying it in any way. This has carried over in other relationships, too. I don't conceal, in the same way, my accomplishments, strengths, etc. and the change feels good."

"With my two children, I am able to differentiate more and treat them separately instead of a 'glob' of two. This is an outgrowth, I feel, of my further differentiating myself from my sisters."

This experience also had impact on her work with client families. She wrote:

"As I have seen how my sisters and I interact, I have become more aware of how members within families that I work with are interacting, i.e., as the fog 'lifts', or I change, I feel that my perception and effectiveness with families increases, to the same degree" (*Family Interfaces*, p. 318).

#11 MALE THERAPIST

"The most significant event was experiencing a sense of rage at a woman group member when she was being helpless and my gradual learning to control and work with it. It was significant because my rage at female helplessness began with my mother and my helplessness to meet my obligation to her. It is frequently present in my relationships with some women, particularly in my family" (*Family Interfaces*, p. 242).

"This insight about my reaction to perceived helplessness has been helpful with my wife and three daughters. At times I perceive all of them as helpless. I am increasingly clear and direct with them and less inclined to help them or feel I ought to all the time."

#12 FEMALE THERAPIST

"I have become aware of how I am following a family pattern by cutting off from certain family members. I am realizing the importance of pushing myself to develop a relationship with each one of those members on a one-to-one basis."

"Since I started changing my relationship with my mother I have been feeling much less depressed. I feel I have finally worked through most of my anger with her. As a result I find I want to be with her; I have more empathy for her and am more sad for what she has been through: I have hopes of becoming a good friend with my mother."

"With my step-daughter, I have become aware of how my fear of being rejected by her (because of rejection by my mother) has kept me distant and protected. I have been able to separate more my relationships with her from my relationship with my mother. There is less contamination. I am able to be more giving with her; I used to get uptight with her demands for my affection and angry at her when she got things I never got. I still get angry sometimes, but am better able to control it, primarily because I understand where it is coming from. It's pretty hard giving to a daughter when your own mother never really knew how to give to you."

DISCUSSION

The effect of working in family training groups on one's own children has not been noted previously in the family therapy literature and particularly not in family therapy training literature. In the follow-up questionnaires done with these groups, the therapists were not asked directly about their children. The statements reported in this paper occurred in the course of a routine follow-up questionnaire. On the one hand, this means that we do not have systematic material, but on the other hand it also shows the importance of these changes, even when they are not focused on.

Explicit differentiation in the relationship with their own children, differentiated from relationships in their families of origin, was mentioned by the eight female and four male therapists, all of whom perceived changes in themselves in relation to their children and, in some cases, in the children themselves. It is interesting to look at the data from these therapists although an analysis does not convey the richness of verbatim material. Summarizing these spontaneous responses is difficult since we recognize that this report is not representative but only a selected sample, and that the perceived changes vary in intensity and in kind.

The female therapists worked on a range of issues which included mother, father, sister, brother, and the more generalized self-family. The male therapists' range was limited to mother and father. The female therapists reported their own changes with 4 sons, 6 daughters, and 2 "children." The male therapists reported changes with 2 sons, 3 daughters, and 2 "kids."

All 12 questionnaires document the therapists' recognition of a connection between their work with their families of origin and their changes in relation to their children, as follows.

For the Female Therapists

#1. Understanding her transference from sister to son allowed her to de-triangle from mother and sister and improve all three relationships.

#2. Recognizing male/female patterns in her family of origin allowed her to give her son more independence, increasing son's feeling of responsibility and self-esteem and decreasing conflict with his sister.

#3. Setting limits in her caretaking of both mother and sister allowed her to take control of her own life and to focus on the needs of her children.

#4. Working out "unfinished business" with brother allowed her to let go of sons so they could learn to take their own consequences for their actions.

#6. Becoming more realistic and accepting of father allowed her to set clear, simple limits with her daughters.

#7. Differentiating from mother allowed her to diminish her protectiveness of son.

#10. Differentiating from sisters allowed her to treat her two children as separate instead of a "glob."

#12. Connecting with her cut-off mother allowed her to separate her relationship with her mother from that with her stepdaughter and to be more giving to her stepdaughter.

Male Therapists

#5. Realizing his own responsibility for his distant relationship with his dead father allowed him to involve himself with his children in new ways.

#8. Taking initiative with father allowed him to permit son to differentiate.

#9. Becoming closer to father and more assertive with mother allowed him to permit son to differentiate.

#11. Controlling rage and recognizing its connection to his helpless feeling with his mother helped him to be increasingly clear and direct and less inclined to see his wife and 3 daughters as helpless.

The report in one of the questionnaires is striking and deserves particular attention (see #3). The female therapist's work with her family of origin, particularly with mother and younger sister, is reflected in the changes in her relationship with her older daughter and also in the daughter herself. She reports increased sensitivity toward this child, who is no longer enuretic and whose childhood asthma has diminished remarkably. With the younger daughter she also reports changes in herself, but not in the child.

SUMMARY

Open ended questionnaires can be used in a number of ways. The result of sifting through family of origin questionnaires for examples of changes with therapists' children gives us a provocative sample which documents, in a tentative way, the connection of changes down through the generations. In-depth studies are indicated.

REFERENCES

Ackerman, N. (1970). Child participation in family therapy. *Family Process*, 9, 403-410.

Bergel, E., Gass, C., & Zilbach, J. (1968). The use of play materials in conjoint therapy. Proceedings of the IVth International Congress of Group Psychotherapy. *Verlag der Weiner Medizinischen Akademie*, 4-16.

Bloch, D.A. (1976). Including the children in family therapy. In P. Guerin (Ed.), *Family Therapy: Theory and Practice* (pp. 168-181). New York: Gardner Press.

Chasin, R. (1981). Involving latency and preschool children in family therapy. In A. Gurman (Ed.), *Questions and Answers in the Practice of Family Therapy*, Vol. I (pp. 32-35). New York: Brunner/Mazel.

Dowling, E., & Jones, H.V.R. (1978). Small children seen and heard in family therapy. *Journal of Child Psychotherapy*, 4 (4), 87-96.

Kramer, J. (1985). *Family Interfaces: Transgenerational Patterns*. New York: Brunner/Mazel.

Zilbach, J. (1982). Young children in family therapy. In A. Gurman (Ed.), *Questions and Answers in the Practice of Family Therapy*, Vol. II. New York: Brunner/Mazel, pp. 65-68.

Zilbach, J., Bergel, E., & Gass, C. (1972). The role of the young child in family therapy. In C. Sager, & H.S. Kaplan (Eds.), *Progress in Group and Family Therapy* (pp. 385-399). New York: Brunner/Mazel.

Zilbach, J. (1986) (with Gordetsky, S. and Brown, D.). *Young Children in Family Therapy*. New York: Brunner/Mazel.

Zilbach, J. (1988). The family life cycle: A framework for understanding children in family therapy. In L. Combrinck-Graham (Ed.), *Children in Family Contexts*. New York: Guilford Press.

RESOURCES

SPECIFIC REFERENCES
ON CHILDREN IN FAMILY THERAPY

Ackerman, N. (1970). Child participation in family therapy. *Family Process*, *9*, 403-410.

Bergel, E., Gass, C., & Zilbach, J. (1968). The use of play materials in conjoint therapy. Proceedings of the IVth International Congress of Group Psychotherapy. *Verlag der Weiner Medizinischen Akadamie*, 4-16.

Bloch, D. A. (1976). Including the children in family therapy. In P. Guerin (Ed.), *Family therapy: Theory and practice*. New York: Gardner Press, pp. 168-181.

Chasin, R. (1981). Involving latency and preschool children in family therapy. In A. Gurman (Ed.), *Questions and answers in the practice of family therapy*, Vol. I. New York: Brunner/ Mazel, pp. 32-35.

Combrinck-Graham, L. (Ed.) (1986). *Treating young children in family therapy*. Rockville, Maryland: Aspen Publishers, Inc.

Combinck-Graham, L. (1988). *Children in Family Contexts*. New York: Guilford Press.

Dowling, E., & Jones, H. V. R. (1978). Small children seen and heard in family therapy. *Journal of Child Psychotherapy*, *4*(4), 87-96.

Gordetsky, S., Zilbach, J., & Bennett, M. (1979, April 1). Child therapy—Its contribution to family therapy. Paper presented at the annual meeting of the American Orthopsychiatric Association.

Guttman, H. (1975). The child's participation in conjoint family therapy. *Journal of the American Academy of Child Psychiatry, 14*, 490-499.

Haley, J. (1973). Strategic therapy when a child is presented as a problem. *Journal of the American Academy of Child Psychiatry, 12*, 641-659.

Levant, R. F., & Haffey, N. A. (1981). Integration of child and family therapy. *International Journal of Family Therapy, 3*(2), 5-10.

Montalvo, B., & Haley, J. (1973). In defense of child therapy. *Family Process, 12*, 227-244.

Scharff, D., & Scharff, J. (1987). *Object relations family therapy*. Chapters 13-15. Northvale, New Jersey: Jason Aronson, Inc., pp. 285-367.

Tiller, J. W. G. (1978). Brief family therapy for childhood tic syndrome. *Family Process, 17*, 217-223.

Villeneuve, C. (1979). The specific participation of the child in family therapy. *Journal of the American Academy of Child Psychiatry, 18*, 44-53.

Zilbach, J. J. (1982). Young children in family therapy. In A. Gurman (Ed.), *Questions and answers in the practice of family therapy*, Vol. II. New York: Brunner/Mazel, pp. 65-68.

Zilbach, J. J. (1986). *Young child in family therapy*. New York: Brunner/Mazel.

Zilbach, J. J., Bergel, E., & Gass, C. (1972). The role of the young child in family therapy. In C. Sager, & H.S. Kaplan (Eds.), *Progress in group and family therapy*. New York: Brunner/Mazel, pp. 385-399.